Register Now for Online Access to Your Book!

SPRINGER PUBLISHING COMPANY
CONNECT™

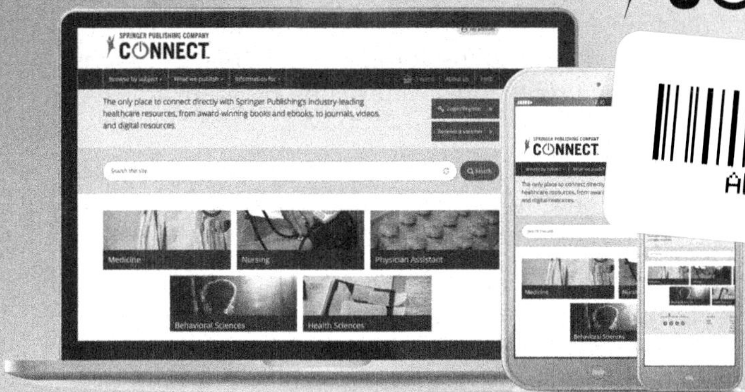

AF708555

Your print purchase of *A Practical Ethics Worktext for Professional Counselors* **includes online access to the contents of your book**—increasing accessibility, portability, and searchability!

Access today at:

http://connect.springerpub.com/content/book/978-0-8261-6534-3 or scan the QR code at the right with your smartphone and enter the access code below.

ESYN7X0T

Scan here for quick access.

If you are experiencing problems accessing the digital component of this product, please contact our customer service department at cs@springerpub.com

The online access with your print purchase is available at the publisher's discretion and may be removed at any time without notice.

Publisher's Note: New and used products purchased from third-party sellers are not guaranteed for quality, authenticity, or access to any included digital components.

SPRINGER PUBLISHING COMPANY

View all our products at springerpub.com

Charles Jacob, PhD, is a lecturer in the Counseling and Mental Health Services Program at the University of Pennsylvania's Graduate School of Education and is licensed as both a counselor and a psychologist. He is also the interim director of the Professional Counseling Program at Seton Hall University.

Diana L. Wildermuth, PhD, NCC, LPC, is an associate professor of practice at Temple University in the Counseling Psychology Program and is licensed as a professional counselor and certified as a professional school counselor.

Ariane Thomas, PsyD, JD, is a lecturer in educational practice in the Counseling and Mental Health Services Program at the University of Pennsylvania's Graduate School of Education and is licensed as a psychologist.

A PRACTICAL ETHICS WORKTEXT FOR PROFESSIONAL COUNSELORS

APPLYING DECISION-MAKING MODELS TO CASE EXAMPLES

Charles Jacob, PhD

Diana L. Wildermuth, PhD, NCC, LPC

Ariane Thomas, PsyD, JD

SPRINGER PUBLISHING COMPANY

Springer Publishing Company, LLC
11 West 42nd Street, New York, NY 10036
www.springerpub.com
connect.springerpub.com/

Acquisitions Editor: Rhonda Dearborn
Compositor: Amnet Systems

ISBN: 978-0-8261-6533-6
ebook ISBN: 978-0-8261-6534-3
DOI: 10.1891/9780826165343

20 21 22 23 / 5 4 3 2 1

Library of Congress Cataloging-in-Publication Data

Names: Jacob, Charles, author. | Wildermuth, Diana L., author. | Thomas, Ariane, author.
Title: A practical ethics worktext for professional counselors : applying decision-making models to case examples / Charles Jacob, Diana L. Wildermuth, Ariane Thomas.
Description: New York, NY : Springer Publishing Company, LLC, [2021] | Includes bibliographical references and index.
Identifiers: LCCN 2019058758 (print) | LCCN 2019058759 (ebook) | ISBN 9780826165336 (paperback) | ISBN 9780826165343 (ebook)
Subjects: MESH: Counseling—ethics | Clinical Decision-Making | Problems and Exercises | Case Reports
Classification: LCC RC455.2.E8 (print) | LCC RC455.2.E8 (ebook) | NLM WM 18.2 | DDC 174.2/9689—dc23
LC record available at https://lccn.loc.gov/2019058758
LC ebook record available at https://lccn.loc.gov/2019058759

Charles Jacob: https://orcid.org/0000-0001-6155-1242
Diana L. Wildermuth: https://orcid.org/0000-0002-9694-9362
Ariane Thomas: https://orcid.org/0000-0003-3625-5542

Printed in the United States of America.

Our sincerest thanks to all the students and clients who have inspired us to do good work.

CONTENTS

PREFACE

I neither know nor think that I know.

—Socrates, in Plato's *Apology*

Knowledge without mileage equals [nothing].

—Henry Rollins

Mentorship is critical to the developing counselor, and I have been fortunate enough to have had some truly gifted supervisors of my clinical work over the years. There are a great many pieces of wisdom I have heard from these folks that were personally meaningful, but a comment from a recent supervisor stands out above all the others: "Counseling is a weird way to make a living." This statement might read as a little cynical, but I know exactly what he meant. He said this not to disparage the profession or the practice of counseling in general; he was merely highlighting that the mix of art and science that goes along with this work can make for some strange moments that require both an openness to ambiguity and a tremendous amount of patience.

Nowhere is this more accurate than with ethics. Though the American Counseling Association (ACA) has offered guidelines for the ethical practice of counseling since 1961, it provides little in the way of definitive answers. The most recent iteration of the Code of Ethics makes clear that ethical decision-making requires thoughtful consideration of myriad variables. The abbreviated list of these considerations includes the values of the profession, its guiding ethical principles and standards, the cultural concerns of the clients being served, and the personal values and beliefs of the counselor. This means that when I, as a counselor, am faced with an ethical dilemma of some kind—say my client is 13 years old and his mother is requesting a copy of his chart—I have to think about and reconcile at least three perspectives:

1. What best serves the profession of counseling? (Should I try to keep all information private, even though his mother is his legal guardian? Isn't confidentiality the cornerstone of good counseling?)

2. What is in the best interest of my client? (If his mom is his legal guardian, maybe there are things in that chart she needs to know for safety reasons—but if I were 13, I would never want to see a counselor who told my mother everything we discussed.)
3. What do *I* want to do? (As a counselor, I definitely do not like the idea of someone's mother reading my clinical notes about his or her child.)

In short, there are few definitive answers, the path to an ethical decision is convoluted at times, and learning to reconcile personal values with professional values can be extremely complicated (see Ametrano, 2014, for a detailed review).

It Depends...

In teaching ethics to counseling students, I have always found that one standard maxim applies when explaining how to manage ethical concerns: *It depends*. At most of the institutions I have taught at over the years, this two-word declaration is often jokingly attached to the faculty tasked with teaching the ethics courses. On more than one occasion in an ethics class I have taught, case example discussions were interrupted with students sarcastically intoning "Wait, let me guess. *It depends*, right?" In some classes, this exchange happened so often it became something of an inside joke (albeit a good-natured one). Ethical codes are written with some degree of ambiguity to allow for flexibility in their application, so it would serve to reason that there might be some amount of frustration both in teaching and in learning ethical decision-making.

Things have gotten even more equivocal as the ACA Code of Ethics now requires evidence of adherence to specific decision-making models when presented with ethical dilemmas, though "no specific ethical decision-making model is always most effective, so counselors are expected to use a credible model of decision making that can bear public scrutiny of its application" (ACA, 2014, p. 3). While this is a sensible approach given the complexity of the decisions counselors face at times, it leaves a great deal of room for interpretation. What models make sense in what cases? How do they apply? If there is a *right* answer, what is it?

The Real World of Clinical Practice Versus the Safety and Security of a Grad School Classroom

I have taught ethics and worked as a clinician long enough to have compiled (what I hope is) an impressive list of ethical quagmires. One of my favorites happened during my internship as a grad student. My doctoral program was in a small town where there were very few gymnasiums and very few mental health facilities. After a morning workout at the gym where I was a member, I showered, walked out into the locker room in nothing but a towel ... and saw three separate clients in various states of undress in the locker room as well.

Obviously, I understood the basics as taught to me in my own graduate program: It is usually best to avoid acknowledging clients in public unless they acknowledge you first. But what about my own sense of privacy here? Further, what do I do now that I know I attend the same gym as three of my clients? In that moment, what can I do that best meets my own personal needs and demonstrates respect for all three clients as well as a commitment to the ethics of my profession? Do I just get dressed and pretend like I don't see them? Run to the bathroom stall and hide until they leave?

This has always been a *crowd favorite* in the classes I have taught, likely as the content is amusing in some way—nothing breaks up the monotony of an ethics lecture like a story about me in a towel. Most of the classes typically spend upward of 10 minutes waxing hypothetical about what they might do if they were in this predicament, what to consider, and what options to contemplate; at which point I stop the discussion and remind them that—in real time—they have been standing in a locker room in their towel, staring into space, for about 10 minutes now.

In class, the point of this anecdote is to begin a dialogue about ethical decision-making as much as it is to highlight the shortcomings of training. When this incident occurred, I had spent what could best be described as a ridiculous amount of time in higher education related to professional counseling, but I was in no way prepared for a situation like this. I also had no time to consult the Code of Ethics or to touch base with my supervisor. All I could do in that moment was hope that I understood the Code, myself, and the needs of my clients well enough to make a good decision in a matter of seconds.

This example also showcases that ethical decision-making in counseling seems to happen in two ways (see Kahneman & Egan, 2011): First, the actual moment where the clinician is faced with a decision and forced to act in some way, and, second, the reasoning, where documentation and justification occur, as counselors are obligated to demonstrate that they followed the appropriate protocol in making the decision that they did. Sometimes you start with reasoning, where the decision is made over days, weeks, or longer, and the action connected to the decision takes less than a second. I once spent an entire afternoon with a supervisor agonizing over the tone of a client's voice message, vacillating between fear for the client's safety and concerns about manipulation, trying to decide if I should return the client's call now or wait until the person came in for the scheduled session. In the case of the locker room incident earlier, I had only a second to make a decision, and the reasoning happened afterward when I outlined my actions in my clinical notes. Whether it happens at the front or the back end of a decision, counselors need to carefully demonstrate the specific steps that led to a specific decision.

How to Use This Book

This book is intended to be used as an addendum to a more comprehensive text associated with the Professional Counseling Orientation and Ethical Practice training required by the Council for Accreditation of Counseling and Related Educational Programs (CACREP, n.d., F.1.a–m). The goal of this text is to provide—as stated in the title—practical examples of managing ethical concerns for practicing counselors and counselors in training. Much has been made of the *science-to-service* problem in counseling (Murray, 2009), with the consensus being that there is a gap between the academics writing the books and papers and the clinicians actually doing the work. This text is an effort to meet the needs of both by providing an overview of case examples that are relatable and accessible and by providing responses to these cases that meet the careful scrutiny required by the ACA.

Chapter Breakdown

Each chapter will include seven cases related to a section of the ACA Code of Ethics examined carefully using a decision-making model.

Chapter 1

ACA Code of Ethics Section: The Counseling Relationship (Section A)
Decision-Making Model: Forester-Miller and Davis (2016)

Cases in this section are all about the relationship between the counselor and the clients. The word *relationship* should be highlighted here, as it denotes a connection between two or more people. This section highlights all the ways in which that connection can become confusing and/or complicated, including, but not limited to, counselors separating personal and professional lives, the tricky business of personal values, and the complexity of boundaries within the counseling relationship.

Chapter 2

ACA Code of Ethics Section: Confidentiality and Privacy (Section B)
Decision-Making Model: Cottone's (2001) Social Constructivist model

Cases in this section deal more specifically with maintaining the confidence and trust of the general public. It is unlikely that counseling could continue to exist as a practice without the public's enduring belief that what is discussed with their counselor remains private. This section highlights some of the unique presenting problems related to confidentiality and privacy, including, but not limited to, seeing clients in public, accidental lapses in confidentiality, requests for information from third parties, and state law pertaining to age and consent.

Chapter 3

ACA Code of Ethics Section: Professional Responsibility (Section C)
Decision-Making Model: Ling and Hauck's (2017) ETHICS Model

The profession of counseling does not exist in a vacuum, and this section details counselors' interactions with the public. Counselors are responsible for presenting the profession (and themselves) to the public in a way that engenders trust and confidence. This section highlights the ways in which counselors' professional responsibility can present both personal and professional challenges, including, but not limited to, responding to peers and supervisors who are impaired in their ability to practice, responding to evidence of malpractice in colleagues, and maintaining professionalism throughout interactions with the public.

Chapter 4

ACA Code of Ethics Section: Relationships With Other Professionals (Section D)
Decision-Making Model: Corey, Corey, and Callanan (2015)

When thinking of ethics in counseling, it can be easy to forget that these criteria extend to our coworkers and office mates as much as they do our clients. Relationships with peers can be surprisingly complicated, but the survival of the profession is predicated on our ability to work collaboratively. This section highlights the complexities of these relationships, including, but not limited to, differences of opinion in client management, staffing concerns, behavior in public, and resolving ethical concerns collaboratively.

Chapter 5

ACA Code of Ethics Section: Evaluation, Assessment, and Interpretation (Section E)
Decision-Making Model: Garcia, Cartwright, Winston, and Borzuchowska's (2003) Transcultural Integrative Model

Testing and evaluation are typically one of the last areas of mental health practice claimed by psychology alone, but assessment is a critical part of work as a counselor. The wellness-focused approach of the profession is in some ways at odds with the labeling required of evaluation, assessment, and interpretation, but these are an undeniable reality of clinical practice in the era of managed care. This section highlights the ways in which assessment in general can become a complex area of practice, including, but not limited to, using diagnosis as a tool for billing, validity of assessment instruments administered to clients, diagnosis and wellness principles, and scope of competence.

Chapter 6

ACA Code of Ethics Section: Supervision, Teaching, and Training (Section F)
Decision-Making Model: Hill, Glaser, and Harden's (1998) Feminist Model

Cases in this section address both the education of counselors in training and the need for lifelong learning as a part of counselor identity. The world of academia can be complex in its efforts to meet the needs of students, faculty, and the public, but practicing clinicians are also expected to stay informed of the science that drives their profession. This section highlights the ethics of supervision, training, and teaching, including, but not limited to, relationships with superiors, values in education and training, the use of case examples, and confidentiality in supervision.

Chapter 7

ACA Code of Ethics Section: Research and Publication (Section G)
Decision-Making Model: Jacob, Roth, Cilento, and Stoler (2015)

While counselors are not required to conduct research as a part of clinical practice, many work in academic settings where scholarship is a regular part of their responsibilities. At the very least, all practicing clinicians should be aware of the ethical responsibilities inherent in the science that governs their work. This section highlights the specific components of ethical counseling research and related complications, including, but not limited to, relationships with participants, credit for work and authorship, and submissions to peer-reviewed outlets.

Chapter 8

ACA Code of Ethics Section: Distance Counseling, Technology, and Social Media (Section H)
Decision-Making Model: Kocet and Herlihy's Counselor Value-Based Conflict Model (2014)

This section was a new addition to the Code of Ethics during its most recent revision in 2014. The advent of technology is unavoidable in all professions, and counseling is no exception. This section highlights the ways in which technological advancements have made counseling both easier and more complicated, including, but not limited to, the use of video conferencing, public and private social media presence, and the importance of safeguarding confidentiality.

Chapter 9

Resolving Ethical Issues (Section I)

Cases in this section will undertake the more *meta* task of using ethical guidelines to govern their adherence to ethical guidelines. No specific decision-making model will be endorsed for this chapter. Instead, the authors select models from previous chapters as applicable to the cases.

Case Breakdown

For each of the 63 cases presented, the following sections will be available to act as an exemplar for how ethical decisions are made or to facilitate group discussions:

Questions for Discussion

For each case, a short list of questions is included to both facilitate insight regarding the presenting concerns and provide a catalyst for group discussion. These questions can be used as either a starting point for an in-class activity or simply as *food for thought* when reading through the text independently. The cases and their interpretations are—of course—subjective, and further discussion based on different interpretation of the presenting concerns is encouraged.

Straight From the Code

Each case has been crafted to correspond to a specific section of the Code, and the specific standards relevant to the case are outlined here. Only the Code of Ethics for the American Counseling Association will be referenced for this book, though discrepancies in other codes (e.g., the American Psychological Association Code of Ethics, the American School Counseling Association Code of Ethics) may be highlighted where relevant. Keep in mind that few cases are addressed completely by one standard alone, so some of these sections will be longer for some cases than for others.

Applying a Decision-Making Model

Chapter 2, Confidentiality and Privacy (Section B of the ACA Code of Ethics), provides a succinct overview of several well-regarded decision-making models for professional counselors. For this section, we take a highly regarded decision-making model for professional counselors and apply it to the presented case. For some of these models, the descriptive process can be quite elaborate, requiring several bullet points and lists to address specific concerns. Please remember that all interpretations of these models are—like the process of ethical decision-making in general—completely subjective.

The Likely Answer

Of all the sections in our text, I encourage you to approach this one with greatest caution. One of the pieces of advice I give to students preparing for licensing exams is that any question pertaining to ethics will likely *not* have a correct answer that is definitive in wording. For example, a correct answer to a multiple-choice ethics question will probably not use wording such as *absolutely*, *definitely*, or *without exception*, as very little in ethics is without ambiguity. As such, remember that the likely answer outlined here is just that: the *likely* (and often completely subjective) answer that the authors were able to piece together using the information and decision-making models presented. Alternative answers are both acceptable and encouraged as a spur for further discussion in groups or consideration independently.

Charles Jacob, PhD

References

American Counseling Association. (2014). *ACA code of ethics.* Alexandria, VA: Author.

Ametrano, I. M. (2014). Teaching ethical decision making: Helping students reconcile personal and professional values. *Journal of Counseling and Development, 92*(2), 154–161. doi:10.1002/j.1556-6676.2014.00143.x

Corey, G., Corey, M. S., Corey, C., & Callanan, P. (2015). *Issues and ethics in the helping professions* (9th ed.). Stamford, CT: Brooks/Cole.

Cottone, R. R. (2001). A social constructivism model of ethical decision-making in counseling. *Journal of Counseling and Development, 79*(1), 39–45. doi:10.1002/j.1556-6676.2001.tb01941.x

Council for Accreditation of Counseling and Related Educational Programs. (n.d.). *What is CACREP?* Retrieved from http://www.cacrep.org

Forester-Miller, H., & Davis, T. E. (2016). *Practitioner's guide to ethical decision-making* (Rev. ed.). Retrieved from https://www.counseling.org/docs/default-source/ethics/practioner-39-s-guide-to-ethical-decision-making.pdf?sfvrsn=10

Garcia, J. G., Cartwright, B., Winston, S. M., & Borzuchowska, B. (2003). A transcultural integrative model for ethical decision-making in counseling. *Journal of Counseling and Development, 81*(3), 268–277. doi:10.1002/j.1556-6678.2003.tb00253.x

Hill, M., Glaser, K., & Harden, J. (1998). A feminist model for ethical decision making. *Women & Therapy, 21*(3), 101–121. doi:10.1300/J015v21n03_10

Jacob, C. J., Roth, G., Cliento, B., & Stoler, J. (2015). The 2014 ACA code of ethics: What's new, what's the same, and what matters for practicing clinicians. *Journal of the Pennsylvania Counseling Association, 14*, 39–46.

Kahneman, D., & Egan, P. (2011). *Thinking, fast and slow* (Vol. 1). New York, NY: Farrar, Straus and Giroux.

Kocet, M. M., & Herlihy, B. J. (2014). Addressing value-based conflicts within the counseling relationship: A decision-making model. *Journal of Counseling and Development, 92*(2), 180–186.

Murray, C. E. (2009). Diffusion of innovation theory: A bridge for the research-practice gap in counseling. *Journal of Counseling and Development, 87*(1), 108–116. doi:10.1002/j.1556-6678.2009.tb00556.x

ACKNOWLEDGMENTS

Special thanks to Anita Das, Nicole Flibbert, Griffin Stockton-Hogrogian, Rebecca Adleberg, and Ben Shaver.

CHAPTER 1

THE COUNSELING RELATIONSHIP (SECTION A OF THE ACA CODE OF ETHICS)

INTRODUCTION

At its most basic, counseling is a relationship, as it involves a connection between two or more people. The following cases outline the ways in which this relationship requires careful thought and planning to ensure the safety of all clients and the integrity of the profession. The scenarios in this section focus on the personal and professional interactions between counselors and their clients.

All cases will be assessed using Forester-Miller and Davis's (2016) seven-step sequence for making an ethical decision.

FORESTER-MILLER AND DAVIS'S ETHICAL DECISION-MAKING MODEL

One of the most widely accepted—not to mention American Counseling Association (ACA) endorsed—approaches to ethical decision-making is Forester-Miller and Davis's ethical decision-making model. A practice-based model, this approach enumerates seven steps that should assist counselors in coming to a reasonable decision regarding ethical dilemmas. The model suggests that counselors:

1. **Identify the problem.** The goal is to identify the nature and scope of the ethical concern(s) presented. Who are the *stakeholders* (clients, clinicians, the general public, the employment setting, etc.) in this particular situation? Are the major concerns connected to law, ethics, or clinical practice?

2. **Apply the ACA Code of Ethics.** Counselors are expected to reference the code either directly in the moment or in the aftermath of decision-making to verify the accuracy of a specific judgment or action. What sections or specific elements of the ACA code apply?

3. **Determine the nature and dimensions of the dilemma.** Specifically, what are the needs of the client, the needs of the profession, and any conflicting needs presented by the clinician(s) in this case? Is there any relevant literature that delineates what should (or should not) happen here? This is also where consultation with experts in the field or with members of the ACA ethics committee and/or state licensing boards may be warranted.

4. **Generate potential courses of action.** This step is all about brainstorming. What might be potential ways to resolve this dilemma? The goal should not be simply to list as many options as possible, but to generate realistic ideas about possible solutions.

5. **Consider the potential consequences of all options and determine a course of action.** For each of the ideas outlined in step 4, what are the potential pros and cons? Based on more careful evaluation of possible outcomes, what ideas can be eliminated from the list determined in step 4?

6. **Evaluate the selected course of action.** For the possible course of action that seems to generate the most benefit and the least harm, how will the counselors be able to determine that a desirable outcome was achieved? Is this decision as fair as possible? Would this outcome be embarrassing to the clinician or the profession in general if it were made public? From the clinician's perspective, is this what they would recommend to anyone else in their situation?

7. **Implement the course of action.** Determine what exactly will be done and how. Clinicians should also follow up in the aftermath of their decisions to determine their efficacy overall.

CONTROLLING FOR BIAS AND PERSONAL VALUES IN COUNSELING (*COUNSELING IS A VALUE-ABLE SERVICE*)

Joseph is a counselor working for a college counseling center at a small Christian university. He has been at this position for just 6 months now and is experiencing some struggles with reconciling his personal values with the values of the institution. Specifically, he identifies as an atheist, but he is regularly reminded of the university's commitment to Christianity and Christian values.

As Joseph's shift is nearing its end at about 4 p.m. on a Friday, a young woman, Mary, comes in for an intake session during "drop-in" hours. As the only counselor available, Joseph agrees to meet with her for an intake session. Midway through this introductory meeting, she begins to cry, stating that she recently found out that she is pregnant and is considering an abortion. She asks him if he can help her "figure out what to do."

Joseph is very aware of his personal bias in this case: He identifies as pro-choice, in that he believes a woman should maintain the individual right to have an abortion if she chooses. However, he has been instructed by his supervisor and other university administrators that all faculty and staff must promote the basic values of Christianity in their counseling. In fact, his supervisor has explicitly stated that he should *not* advocate anything that is not "explicitly aligned with the church's values," including abortion.

Questions for Discussion

1. *How will Joseph account for his personal values in a way that does not have an impact on counseling?*
2. *If the values of his employer are not in line with the values of the counseling profession, what should Joseph do?*
3. *Is it acceptable for Joseph to offer any direct advice in this situation?*

Straight From the Code

1. **A.4.b. Personal Values.** Counselors are aware of, and avoid imposing, their own values, attitudes, beliefs, and behaviors. Counselors respect the diversity of clients, trainees, and research participants and seek training in areas in which they are at risk of imposing their values onto clients, especially when the counselor's values are inconsistent with the client's goals or are discriminatory in nature.

Applying a Decision-Making Model: Forester-Miller and Davis's Ethical Decision-Making Model

1. **Identify the problem.** The primary problem is that a conflict exists among Joseph's values, the values of the institution where he is employed, and, to some extent, the values of the counseling profession. Joseph believes that Mary should be able to have an abortion if she chooses, but he needs to be sure that he does not allow this value to skew the intervention or support he provides. The university believes that Mary should *not* be able to have an abortion and that Joseph should refrain from any indication, through direct guidance or by refusing to provide direct guidance, that suggests otherwise. Finally, the values of the counseling profession seem to suggest that Mary should have the autonomy to make whatever choice she feels is in her best interest, regardless of the beliefs of her counselor or the university she attends.

2. **Apply the ACA Code of Ethics.** This section of the code (A) is clear that counselors should not impose their own values on their clients. The code also indicates that counselors should avoid discriminating against clients where religion is concerned (C.5) and are obligated to accept the policies of any institution where they are employed (D.1.g.). They should, however, alert employers when policies are inappropriate or potentially harmful to clients (D.1.h.).

3. **Determine the nature and dimensions of the dilemma.** One of the major areas of concern is how Joseph should handle a discrepancy between the ethics of the profession and the values of his employer. If

he tacitly supports Mary's decision to have an abortion and the university finds out, he could lose his job. If Joseph imposes the will of the university by suggesting to his client that it is against the rules of the Church to have an abortion, he is violating his own values and refusing to allow his client autonomy.

It should be noted that the institution in this case has the right to promote and uphold whatever values it chooses. Christian universities reserve the right to promote a specific mission that contains specific values (see Bryn Athyn College, 2019), and the university's refusal to condone abortion is not necessarily a violation of student rights.

4. **Generate potential courses of action.** One possible option would be to simply listen to Mary as she navigates this dilemma, providing support and refraining from offering any specific direction. This is likely in keeping with the humanistic fundamentals of the profession (e.g., Wampold, 2012), though it may contradict the values of the institution. If so, Joseph could follow up by bringing this to the attention of his supervisors, as it may be important for them to understand that counseling requires clients be granted autonomy. It might be helpful to work toward negotiating a change in policy regarding the regulations applicable to the counseling center if possible.

   Joseph could also allow Mary the space to go over her own list of possible choices but reiterate to her that as an employee of an institution committed to Christian values, he could not explicitly advocate that she have an abortion. He could highlight to her that while this particular stance is not in keeping with the values of professional counseling, it is the rule in place at their university.

5. **Consider the potential consequences of all options and determine a course of action.** If Joseph decides on the first option (to simply listen to Mary as she navigates this dilemma, providing support and refraining from offering any specific direction), he should likely follow up with his supervisor immediately to outline his concerns and to see if any institutional change is possible. If so, he should advocate that a counselor's role is not to direct people in any choice but to allow them the freedom to explore all options available. If the university refuses to agree to this, Joseph will have to make a difficult decision between keeping his job and adhering to his own values. If the institution decides that anything less than a pro-life stance is unacceptable, they are likely within their right to do so.

   If Joseph decides on the second option (to allow Mary the space to explore her options but also reminding her of the values of the institution), this reminder may serve as little more than a disclaimer about the values of the institution. Joseph will need to carefully monitor the delivery of his statement (e.g., is he saying it in a way that indicates he believes it, or does it sound like he disagrees?) to ensure that it serves only as a reminder and is not intended to steer her in any particular direction. He should use this same caution in allowing Mary to explore the extent to which her own values affect her decision-making process, particularly to ensure that his pro-choice beliefs are kept in check.

6. **Evaluate the selected course of action.** Of the two options, transparency with the institution seems to be the better course of action. If Joseph can run this situation past his supervisor and superiors at the university, there is a good chance of advocating for the profession of counseling in an important way. This would also provide him the possibility of engaging in the second option during a future session if his employer enforces this value as a requirement for employment.

7. **Implement the course of action.** This situation is likely to create a number of challenging conversations, particularly if it requires Joseph to discuss policies with his supervisors and administrators within the university. Difficult conversations are never fun (especially when they involve topics as heavy as employment and religious values), but this might be a necessary course of action if the university's policies affect all individuals receiving help at the university counseling center.

The Likely Answer

As stated earlier, Joseph should do his best to be supportive, allow Mary to talk out all possible options, and then go to his supervisor immediately to outline the contradiction between the university and the counseling profession to see what can be negotiated.

PERSONAL VIRTUAL RELATIONSHIPS WITH CLIENTS (*FACEBOOK-ING YOUR FEARS*)

Annaliese is a counselor at a drug and alcohol clinic in an urban area. She has been seeing Tim for individual and group counseling for the past 3 months as part of an intensive outpatient program for alcohol dependency. For Tim, the support provided by Annaliese during his stepdown from inpatient detox has been "nothing short of invaluable," and he is now preparing to step down to the next level of care (weekly individual counseling with an outpatient provider).

During their last individual session, Tim again says how valuable Annaliese's support has been and expresses an interest in maintaining contact. He is a musician and is excited to get back to performing with his band, a rock and electronic group named Dekkar, which he regularly discussed as one of the most important things in his life during their meetings.

Tim asks Annaliese if she would be willing to follow his band on social media using her Facebook page. He promises not to try to connect with her using his own personal Facebook page but states that it would "mean a lot" if he knew she checked out his music.

Questions for Discussion

1. *Are social connections of any kind appropriate with former clients?*
2. *Is Tim's proposed connection appropriate as it is a request to follow an artist page (as opposed to a personal page)?*
3. *If Annaliese opts to deny his request, can she do so without hurting Tim's feelings?*

Straight From the Code

1. **A.5.e. Personal Virtual Relationships With Current Clients.** Counselors are prohibited from engaging in a personal virtual relationship with individuals with whom they have a current counseling relationship (e.g., through social and other media).
2. **A.6.e. Nonprofessional Interactions or Relationships (Other Than Sexual or Romantic Interactions or Relationships).** Counselors should avoid entering into nonprofessional relationships with former clients, their romantic partners, or their family members when the interaction is potentially harmful to the client. This applies to both in-person and electronic interactions or relationships.

Applying a Decision-Making Model: Forester-Miller and Davis's Ethical Decision-Making Model

1. **Identify the problem.** In this case, the problem is relatively simple: Tim is attempting to maintain a personal relationship with Annaliese after treatment has ended. Though his overture is connected to his interest in music, the description clearly indicates that Tim has expressed an interest in "maintaining contact."
2. **Apply the ACA Code of Ethics.** The code appears to be very straightforward with matters such as these: Virtual relationships are to be avoided both during treatment (A.5.e.) and after treatment has concluded (A.6.e.). It should be noted, however, that the wording for both is slightly different: While virtual relationships with current clients are "prohibited," relationships with former clients are to be "avoid[ed]."
3. **Determine the nature and dimensions of the dilemma.** The main concern here is that while Tim is no longer an active client, denying his request could potentially cause him emotional hurt. This is in no

way guaranteed, but how to tactfully deny unwanted friend requests on social media has been a cause of great discomfort for many since its inception (Baum, 2010). The concern is that anytime a person expresses an interest in a social connection that is denied, the rejection creates a potential to offend or hurt.

4. **Generate potential courses of action.** One option would be for Annaliese to simply cite the code of ethics, stating that social media connections of any kind with former clients are to be avoided. Another option would be for her to interpret a connection through an artist page as something other than a relationship and to accept this request on the contingency that it go no further.

5. **Consider the potential consequences of all options and determine a course of action.** If Annaliese decides to reject this request by way of directly citing the code, she still risks the chance of offending or harming a client that is being discharged following a recent struggle with substance abuse. If she opts to accept this request, she will publicly express interest in a former client's social media, which the code (at the very least) indicates is to be avoided. Were a colleague or supervisor to become aware of this, it is unlikely that it would result in anything as severe as the loss of her license, but Annaliese should likely consult the relevant employee handbook(s) or related literature available through her place of employment. Also, this creates a problem for future counseling for Annaliese and Tim. If Tim returns to her for treatment in a few months' time, her connection to him through social media has now shifted from ethically questionable to something the code states is "forbidden."

6. **Evaluate the selected course of action.** Of the two options, the risk of offense to the client seems to bring about the lesser possibility of harm overall. If Tim is unable to accept that this type of interaction is inappropriate as outlined in the code of ethics, it may be an indication that, as he stated in the initial request, this is less about sharing his art and more about maintaining a connection with his former counselor.

7. **Implement the course of action.** If Annaliese is able to respond to Tim in the moment, she can directly tell him no and cite the code as one reason why and the importance of keeping a return to treatment as a potential option as another. If the request comes in writing by way of a social media message, she can say the same thing in a short, polite missive.

The Likely Answer

Annaliese should politely say no, keep the door open for future counseling sessions as needed, and revisit boundary issues if Tim returns (also as needed).

CONFIDENTIALITY IN GROUP COUNSELING (*WHOOPS! WRONG ROOM*)

Mildred is a counselor who has managed her own private practice for the past 10 years where she sees mostly adolescent clients for individual counseling. As business has been struggling the past year or so, she has been exploring other options for potential income. At the recommendation of a colleague, Mildred has started a weekly counseling support group for young women, which has been running successfully for the past month. Most of the members are referrals from other mental health professionals in the area, but a few members are clients that Mildred also sees individually.

During a recent group session, one of her individual/group clients, G.G., reports to the group that she has been struggling with trust in her relationship with her boyfriend and talks for a bit about her struggles with anxiety. The group, in general, is supportive, but G.G. begins to cry when discussing some of her stress and frustration related to intimacy. Mildred offers support as well, stating that she is impressed with G.G.'s capacity for strength and resilience, particularly in light of her past history of sexual abuse as a child.

At this last statement, G.G. looks horrified, and the rest of the group seems equal parts confused and surprised. Mildred immediately realizes that G.G. had shared this with her in individual counseling and *not* with the group.

Questions for Discussion

1. *What should Mildred do in this moment to mollify what has happened? Should she admit what has happened to the group?*
2. *Has Mildred violated any basic ethical principles by seeing a client for both group and individual counseling at the same time?*
3. *How will Mildred reestablish trust such that individual counseling can continue with G.G.?*

Straight From the Code

1. **A.9.a. Screening.** Counselors screen prospective group counseling/therapy participants. To the extent possible, counselors select members whose needs and goals are compatible with the goals of the group, who will not impede the group process, and whose well-being will not be jeopardized by the group experience.

2. **A.9.b. Protecting Clients.** In a group setting, counselors take reasonable precautions to protect clients from physical, emotional, or psychological trauma.

Applying a Decision-Making Model: Forester-Miller and Davis's Ethical Decision-Making Model

1. **Identify the problem.** The primary problem is that Mildred has accidentally divulged personal information to a group of individuals without the client's consent. A secondary concern is whether it is appropriate for Mildred to see clients for both individual and group counseling concurrently.

2. **Apply the ACA Code of Ethics.** The decision to see clients for both individual and group work is not specifically supported or prohibited in the code, though addressing the changing nature of relationships within counseling is discussed in section A.6.d. Mildred should have screened her potential participants carefully (particularly her current individual clients) to make sure that there were no concerns that would jeopardize the group or individuals' well-being.

   How to screen for this kind of information is a difficult question to address. What constitutes such concerns (e.g., compatible needs, will not impede the group process) is unclear and may vary from setting to setting or client to client. In the case of a basic support group for adolescents, it seems unlikely that G.G.'s history of abuse would have in any way precluded her from attending in the first place. However, counselors who decide to see clients in individual and group settings concurrently should at the very least discuss these potential concerns as part of informed consent and throughout treatment.

3. **Determine the nature and dimensions of the dilemma.** Though screening participants may or may not have been a dilemma initially, the concern at present is how to handle the slip of information that has occurred. Mildred may have been in the right to see G.G. in both settings, but the primary concern at the moment is that information that a client did not consent to be released has been disclosed in a group setting.

4. **Generate potential courses of action.** One possible option would be to address the breach immediately within the group setting. The group as a whole appears aware of what has happened, and it may be unavoidable to process this in the moment. Another option might be to "table" discussion of the incident until Mildred is able to meet privately with G.G. to determine how she would like to handle the matter.

5. **Consider the potential consequences of all options and determine a course of action.** If Mildred decides on the first option, processing the incident in the moment, she is addressing the concern as it occurs in the present, which seems ideal in some ways. It seems that both the group and G.G. are aware of what has happened in this moment,

and to push ahead without addressing what has happened would be questionable. This would require Mildred to openly admit fault to the group as a whole, as she would need to first indicate that she accidentally betrayed the confidence of a group member, and then ask G.G. how she would like to proceed.

If Mildred decides on the second option—to table discussion of the incident until she is able to meet with G.G. privately—she runs the risk of damaging rapport with the entire group. While this may allow G.G. the opportunity to make a more informed decision about how to handle the matter, it would likely be complicated to continue the group without discussing what is both an obvious error on behalf of the leader and a compelling disclosure about one of its members.

6. **Evaluate the selected course of action.** Of the two basic options, processing the incident in the moment seems inevitable. Mildred will have to determine how to proceed with this course of action in a way that affords respect to both the group and G.G. She could begin by addressing the incident outright, admitting that she clearly just made a disclosure accidentally, apologize to both G.G. and to the group overall, and then ask G.G. how she would like to proceed.

7. **Implement the course of action.** In doing so, Mildred will have to be willing to accept that both G.G. and the group could be angry at her for what has happened. Her slip up was an honest mistake, and even with appropriate screening of group members, it may not have been avoided. It is to be hoped that Mildred had informed group members of the risks inherent in seeing individuals in two settings and that she did not guarantee that missteps would never occur.

The Likely Answer

Mildred needs to pause, admit she made a mistake, process it with G.G. and the group, and meet with G.G. afterward to see what she needs moving forward.

COMPETENCE AND VALUES WITHIN TERMINATION AND REFERRALS (*WHY DIDN'T YOU TELL ME THAT IN THE FIRST PLACE?*)

Petra is a counselor who manages her own private practice. She has been seeing a client, Dylan, for the past 3 months to help him cope with social difficulties and related anxiety. The two have a good rapport, though treatment goals have been difficult to define.

At the start of today's session, Dylan appears nervous. He says that he needs to be honest with Petra about what brought him to treatment in the first place and that he is worried about how she will respond. Petra assures him that she will do her best to be supportive and reminds him that her role as a counselor is to promote respect for human dignity and diversity. Dylan responds by stating that he, a 39-year-old male, has been attracted sexually to young boys for as long as he can remember. He states that he has not acted on these impulses and has no intention of doing so but that he could not continue with counseling if he did not bring this into the discussion. He tells Petra that she has seemed supportive and kind, and he was worried that she would judge him if he told her all of this initially.

Petra is distressed upon hearing this. In addition to being the mother of two young boys herself, Petra has counseled many children and adults who were the victims of childhood sexual abuse. She has training in cognitive behavioral therapy (CBT) for sexual dysfunctions, but she worries that she cannot continue treatment with Dylan as she is strongly biased against individuals who identify as being sexually attracted to children.

Questions for Discussion

1. *Is it acceptable to refer a client out to other providers when a counselor's ability to be objective is potentially compromised?*
2. *Is Petra competent to treat an individual who self-identifies as being attracted to young boys? Is her CBT training sufficient?*
3. *If Petra does continue to treat Dylan, how will she keep her own biases in check?*

Straight From the Code

1. **A.11.a. Competence Within Termination and Referral.** If counselors lack the competence to be of professional assistance to clients, they avoid entering or continuing counseling relationships. Counselors are knowledgeable about culturally and clinically appropriate referral resources and suggest these alternatives. If clients decline the suggested referrals, counselors discontinue the relationship.

2. **A.11.b. Values Within Termination and Referral.** Counselors refrain from referring prospective and current clients based solely on the counselor's personally held values, attitudes, beliefs, and behaviors. Counselors respect the diversity of clients and seek training in areas in which they are at risk of imposing their values onto clients, especially when the counselor's values are inconsistent with the client's goals or are discriminatory in nature.

Applying a Decision-Making Model: Forester-Miller and Davis's Ethical Decision-Making Model

1. **Identify the problem.** The primary problem is that Petra feels uncomfortable on a personal level working with Dylan, now that he has

disclosed his paraphilia. Her competence may be in question as well, as she indicates having training in sexual dysfunction but not paraphilias specifically.

2. **Apply the ACA Code of Ethics.** The code permits termination and referral for issues of competence, but not for conflicts of values. Petra can refer Dylan to a separate provider if she determines her decision is motivated by a lack of sufficient training or experience to provide a specific treatment that is required. If, however, she believes her actions are motivated by personal bias, Petra is obligated to seek support through additional training or supervision.

   Competence is difficult to define, though Petra could likely contend that her training in CBT for sexual dysfunction, while not an indication of expertise, is sufficient enough to qualify as competence. Treatment for pedophilia typically focuses on relapse prevention, with CBT having some support for its ability to reduce recidivism (Lösel & Schmucker, 2005).

3. **Determine the nature and dimensions of the dilemma.** Another problem is that, in this case, the line between competence and value is decidedly thin. If Petra did choose to refer Dylan to another provider, could she say with absolute certainty that this was in his best interest and not a function of her own needs and values? Or can she justify her decision by suggesting that her values would have led to a concern of competence? Assuming the latter, can Petra have personal values that are not in accordance with the ACA?

4. **Generate potential courses of action.** Depending on how she actually feels, Petra could likely validate either continuing with treatment or referring to another provider. Regarding the decision to refer out, she could argue that she has training in CBT but that she is not experienced enough in the treatment of paraphilias to be of help to Dylan. Regarding the decision to continue treatment, she could certainly justify continuing treatment while obtaining additional training or supervision from a mental health professional with greater experience in the treatment of sexual attraction to children.

5. **Consider the potential consequences of all options and determine a course of action.** If Petra decides to continue treatment, she would need to offer Dylan the option of seeking treatment from another provider with greater experience. The decision to continue treatment would need to be made by the client once Petra clearly explains what options are available (i.e., to stay with a provider with less experience with whom he feels connected, or to transfer to a provider with more experience where he will essentially be restarting treatment). She would also have to make clear (and follow through on) her efforts to continue with training and supervision necessary to provide

competent treatment. Petra will likely have to work closely with a clinical supervisor throughout this process to ensure that treatment is in no way seriously compromised by her beliefs and biases.

If Petra instead decides that her competence is in question such that she risks harming Dylan, she should clearly outline why she is unable to continue treatment with him and provide referrals to providers that are within reason both financially and geographically. This in and of itself may prove to be problematic given the social stigma among mental health professionals in the United States attached to sexual attraction to children (Jahnke, Philipp, & Hoyer, 2015), as providers willing to take the referral may be few and far between. Petra will also have to consider that the decision to refer to a separate provider may cause harm to Dylan. If the implicit message from this encounter is that the counselor was uncomfortable with Dylan's presenting concerns, he may be unlikely to seek treatment from another clinician or be less inclined to engage in an honest discussion of his problem in the future.

6. **Evaluate the selected course of action.** Unless Petra honestly believes that she lacks competence to treat Dylan, she seems to have little choice but to continue with treatment at this time. The ACA's decision to discourage referrals based on personal values has received some criticism (see Herlihy, Hermann, & Greden, 2014 for a detailed review), but is ultimately grounded in counseling's humanistic roots. If Petra refuses to treat Dylan, she could be causing him harm, and counselors are obligated to refrain from discrimination of any kind in their clinical practice.

7. **Implement the course of action.** As stated earlier, Petra will have to seek additional training if she feels this is required, but she will, at the very least, need to process these concerns in clinical supervision.

The Likely Answer

We cannot choose who we treat. While the counseling profession does not say that Petra *has* to work with Dylan, it seems clear that she probably *should*.

RECEIVING GIFTS (*FOR ME? HOW LOVELY*)

Kathy is a newly hired school counselor working in a suburban high school. This is her first counseling job after graduate school. She has a caseload of approximately 350 students, ninth to 12th grade. She has been meeting with all the seniors assigned to her to assist with career and college planning. The students seem to like Kathy overall, with many describing her as the "cool young counselor, who gets it."

Kathy has met with Juan, a 19-year-old Latino male senior, several times to assist with college and scholarship applications. Juan's parents were born in Mexico, and he is the first in the family to be born in the United States. His parents do not speak English, and Juan spends most of his summers in Mexico with other family members. The relationship between Kathy and Juan has remained professional but close; she sees him as a student with a lot of potential, and they have spent a lot of time together discussing his plans for the future, speaking about his resultant anxieties, and completing the necessary paperwork to complete Juan's college and scholarship applications.

During one of their final meetings before the summer, Juan tells Kathy that if he gets into college, he will buy her flowers and take her on a date after graduation. Kathy assumes he is joking and laughs it off.

Just before graduation, Juan sends Kathy a bouquet of flowers to her home address. The flowers come with a handwritten note containing a poem written by Juan, wherein he expresses a deep, profound appreciation of Kathy. She is at once both flattered by the sentiment and a little uncomfortable, as the poem has an almost romantic tone.

Questions for Discussion

1. *Should Kathy accept the flowers? Will this hurt the relationship if Kathy does not accept the flowers?*
2. *Would the decision-making process be different if this had occurred in a private practice or clinical mental health setting?*
3. *How will Kathy continue the relationship (if she does, or does not accept the flowers)?*

Straight From the Code

1. **A.5.a. Sexual and/or Romantic Relationships Prohibited.** Sexual and/or romantic counselor–client interactions or relationships with current clients, their romantic partners, or their family members are prohibited. This prohibition applies to both in person and electronic interactions or relationships.

2. **A.10.f. Receiving Gifts.** Counselors understand the challenges of accepting gifts from clients and recognize that in some cultures, small gifts are a token of respect and gratitude. When determining whether to accept a gift from clients, counselors take into account the therapeutic relationship, the monetary value of the gift, the client's motivation for giving the gift, and the counselor's motivation for wanting to accept or decline the gift.

Applying a Decision-Making Model: Forester-Miller and Davis's Ethical Decision-Making Model

1. **Identify the problem.** It seems evident that Juan has a different perception of his relationship with Kathy and that she is obviously uncomfortable with his overture. At the same time, he is showing

gratitude for the help and support Kathy has provided, and there may need to be some consideration of cultural contextual factors.

Obviously, it is unacceptable for Kathy to engage in a romantic relationship with a former client. However, as a new counselor, Kathy may be unsure of what her school's policy is for accepting gifts. In some schools, it may be common practice for students to give teachers gifts during the holidays or at the end of the school year as a token of appreciation. The problem in this case is predominantly connected to how the gift was presented and the way in which Kathy should respond.

2. **Apply the ACA Code of Ethics.** Per the American School Counselor Association (ASCA) ethical code, there is nothing that states a school counselor cannot accept gifts, so referring to ACA is the best first course of action. The ACA code is clear that romantic relationships are wholly inappropriate, but the language regarding gifts is more equivocal. What constitutes a "small" gift is unclear, and the motivations behind accepting or receiving are also hazy. Does a $20 bouquet of flowers meet the criteria for "small?" Does the romantic flavor of the attached poem sully the intentions of the flowers such that accepting them would be inappropriate?

   Context needs to be considered in this case as well. Kathy should refer to the school board policy, as many institutions may have protocols in place that are more direct than what the ACA code outlines. Also, in some cultures, it is disrespectful to not accept a gift. It is expected that Kathy had training as part of her graduate program in working with diverse populations and knows the cultural norms related to receiving gifts, but the individual context that Juan presents needs to be considered carefully.

3. **Determine the nature and dimensions of the dilemma.** The core issue here is whether Kathy should accept or decline the gift and how (or if) to address this with the client moving forward. In consideration of nonmaleficence, Kathy may be concerned that declining the gift could cause more harm than benefit. However, the gift's romantic overtones bring into question Juan's motivations.

4. **Generate potential courses of action.** One option would be for Kathy to accept the flowers, tell Juan "Thank you" when she sees him next, and have that be the end of it. Another option would be to set up a meeting with Juan to discuss and process what has occurred and establish what constitutes acceptable boundaries in their interactions moving forward.

5. **Consider the potential consequences of all options and determine a course of action.** If Kathy accepts the flowers without comment, there are concerns regarding both what Juan will interpret from this action

and what other students in the school or faculty will think. If Kathy responds with a scheduled meeting and review of intentions and protocol, she may embarrass Juan and hurt his feelings.

6. **Evaluate the selected course of action.** Of the two options, simply discussing the gift with Juan seems to make the most sense. It is to be hoped that Kathy has established enough of a rapport with Juan such that a discussion such as this would be possible.
7. **Implement the course of action.** While the selected course of action might be a difficult conversation to have with Juan, it would potentially create further problems if Juan left the counseling relationship with a profound misunderstanding about its parameters. Maintaining a person-centered approach may help facilitate this conversation, and hopefully, it can be done without tremendous hurt on Juan's end.

The Likely Answer

Kathy should accept the flowers (to send them back would likely be impractical), talk to her direct supervisor, review the school's policy, and then ask to talk with Juan about the importance of professional boundaries in counseling (and school), be it with her or with any other counselor he sees moving forward.

ABANDONMENT AND CLIENT NEGLECT WITH TERMINATION (*ALOHA CLIENTS*)

Wendy is a licensed professional counselor in private practice with a caseload of approximately 40 clients. Overall, the practice is a financial success! A few of her clients have been in treatment for over a year (e.g., some attend session weekly, others monthly), and she has scheduled three new client intakes for next week.

It is the Friday before a holiday weekend, and Wendy's partner has just surprised her with an anniversary gift: a vacation to Hawaii for 4 weeks! The flight leaves in 2 days.

Wendy has taken extended vacations before, but never with this short of notice. In the past, she would let her clients know at least a month in advance and would provide all of them with names of colleagues to contact in an emergency during her absence. For current clients, Wendy would do this in person at an appointment where they could discuss a plan of care while she is out of the office. For clients who she had not seen in some time, she would mail a letter to each with detailed information of who to contact in her absence.

Wendy is worried that she will not be able to contact all her clients over the weekend. More so, she is also concerned that she will be unable to find a colleague to fill in while she is away on such short notice.

Questions for Discussion

1. *Is it ever okay to just abandon a practice?*
2. *Can Wendy find a way to meet the needs of her clients without missing an opportunity to enjoy a surprise vacation with her partner?*
3. *Is there anything Wendy can do to prevent something like this from happening in the future?*

Straight From the Code

1. **A.12. Abandonment and Client Neglect.** Counselors do not abandon or neglect clients in counseling. Counselors assist in making appropriate arrangements for the continuation of treatment, when necessary, during interruptions such as vacations, illness, and following termination.

2. **A.11.c. Appropriate Termination**. Counselors terminate a counseling relationship when it becomes reasonably apparent that the client no longer needs assistance, is not likely to benefit, or is being harmed by continued counseling. Counselors may terminate counseling when in jeopardy of harm by the client or by another person with whom the client has a relationship, or when clients do not pay fees as agreed upon. Counselors provide pretermination counseling and recommend other service providers when necessary.

Applying a Decision-Making Model: Forester-Miller and Davis's Ethical Decision-Making Model

1. **Identify the problem.** All counselors deserve a break, and Wendy is no exception. However, she did not know of this vacation, or she would have started to prepare her clients in the past month. The concern is clearly related to Wendy's obligations as a practicing counselor and not abandoning, neglecting, or terminating her clients without notice. Wendy has 2 days over a holiday weekend to figure out who will be the on-call counselor and how she will get this information to each of her clients and the three new ones scheduled for intakes.

2. **Apply the ACA Code of Ethics.** Counselors do not leave or terminate the counselor–client relationship without making arrangements in their absence or providing pretermination counseling, respectively. Since there are potential new clients scheduled, Wendy may also need to consider transferring these cases to a new counselor.

3. **Determine the nature and dimensions of the dilemma.** Wendy needs to act with fidelity and honor the appointments and obligations made

to current and potential clients. She is also entitled to a vacation to practice self-care and reduce burnout.

This example details a vacation, but emergencies occur, and counselors are at times placed in positions where they are incapable of honoring the needs of their clients. If, instead of a vacation, Wendy had suddenly needed to go out of state to care for a sick relative, the problem would be more or less the same. However, the nature of the dilemma is still important to consider. Specifically, if one of her clients were to make a complaint to a licensing board, a sick family member would likely garner more sympathy than a spontaneous luxury vacation.

4. **Generate potential courses of action.** One option would be to simply reach out to all of her clients via phone and inform them that she will need to reschedule their appointments 4 weeks out. In this case, Wendy would also need to provide contact information for another practicing clinician, emergency support numbers (e.g., a 24-hour crisis hotline), and be certain to document this in all of her clients' charts. Another option would be to refuse the vacation out of concern for her clients' well-being.

5. **Consider the potential consequences of all options and determine a course of action.** If Wendy chooses to go, it is unlikely that she would meet the criteria for abandonment, as she is only leaving for a set period of time. However, if something were to happen to one of her clients (e.g., an increase in depression followed by a suicide attempt) that led to an inquiry of some kind, Wendy would have to admit that she left her clients suddenly for an entire month to take a last-minute vacation to Hawaii. If she chooses not to go, she is acting in the best interest of her practice, but this may have an impact on her relationship with her partner.

6. **Evaluate the selected course of action.** Life happens, and it is expected that counselors may have to take leaves of absence for unexpected reasons. If Wendy can quickly determine the needs of her clients, provide appropriate support in her absence, and contact all of them in the brief window available, she can probably go on her vacation.

7. **Implement the course of action.** It looks as if Wendy is going to have a busy weekend making phone calls to all of her clients and checking in with other therapists in the area who can provide support in her absence.

The Likely Answer

As suggested earlier, Wendy needs to sit down, determine the needs of her clients, provide referrals to practicing clinicians in her absence, contact all of her clients, and remind her partner never to do anything like this again without consulting her first.

EXTENDING COUNSELING BOUNDARIES (*BE MY GUEST!*)

Jill has been a high school counselor for the past 12 years in the same school district in a small, tight-knit community. She has gotten to know many students and their families in the district over the years. She currently has a caseload of approximately 300 students, and she is the only high school counselor on staff.

One student on her caseload is a 10th grader named Tim who has been to the counseling office with some concerns about his family and how his older sister Marney has been "getting all the attention" with her upcoming wedding to her fiancé, Steve. Tim has always felt as though he was "in his sister's shadow" and that this wedding is just another example of his family showing preference for her over him. The stress overall has caused him a lot of anxiety and depression, and he has been meeting with Jill regularly for the past year.

To make matters more complicated, Jill was also Marney's counselor when she was a student at the same high school 10 years ago. Marney was a top student in her class, involved in countless activities, and voted class president (twice), and everyone liked her. She saw Jill on and off during her senior year for stress related to college applications. Though Jill is not one to rank her clients according to her personal preferences, she would be lying to herself if she said she did not find Marney to be one of her favorite clients ever.

Out of the blue, Jill receives an invitation to Marney and Steve's wedding in 2 months—she apparently had a greater impact on Marney than she realized! She wants very much to go but knows that this would likely be upsetting to Tim. Tim has not told his family that he sees Jill for counseling, and he would likely be offended to see Jill celebrating the wedding that has annoyed him so thoroughly these past few months.

Questions for Discussion

1. *Can Jill go to the wedding since she is no longer Marney's school counselor? Should she buy a gift or give money?*
2. *If Jill goes to the wedding, should she acknowledge Tim?*
3. *How will Jill continue the relationship with Tim (if she does or does not go to the wedding)?*

Straight From the Code

1. **A.6.b. Extending Counseling Boundaries.** Counselors consider the risks and benefits of extending current counseling relationships

beyond conventional parameters. Examples include attending a client's formal ceremony (e.g., a wedding/commitment ceremony or graduation), purchasing a service or product provided by a client (excepting unrestricted bartering), and visiting a client's ill family member in the hospital. In extending these boundaries, counselors take appropriate professional precautions such as informed consent, consultation, supervision, and documentation to ensure that judgment is not impaired and no harm occurs.

Applying a Decision-Making Model: Forester-Miller and Davis's Ethical Decision-Making Model

1. **Identify the problem.** Jill is conflicted as she wants to go to the wedding but knows that this could have an impact on Tim's treatment and well-being. She is concerned that if she attends the wedding, it will make Tim feel uncomfortable, both because it may identify him as a client in counseling and because it may have an impact on their development or maintenance of rapport.

2. **Apply the ACA Code of Ethics.** As a certified school counselor, Jill should also consult the American School Counselor Association's (ASCA) 2016 Code of Ethics for best practice. She should also refer to school board policy; however, most school districts do not have policies that pertain to attending weddings. In applying the code A.6.b. Extending Counseling Boundaries, Jill is considering attending the wedding and whether to give a gift. She is also considering the complexity of this situation since she is Tim's current counselor. The code does not provide clear guidance in this situation; it only acknowledges that such actions are not outside the realm of acceptable ethical behaviors.

3. **Determine the nature and dimensions of the dilemma.** The core concern is not just whether Jill should go to the wedding but also how this will impact her relationship with Tim. It is important to consider the principle of nonmaleficence. Specifically, Tim appears to be struggling more than his sister, and attending the wedding may cause harm to Tim. However, not going to the wedding could cause harm to Marney, as it may be seen as a betrayal from a trusted former counselor (though this appears unlikely based on the information provided so far).

4. **Generate potential courses of action.** Jill could meet with Tim and discuss her concerns. She could attend the wedding, in which case she might also consider if buying a gift is appropriate. She could also simply decide not to go and send a gift instead.

5. **Consider the potential consequences of all options and determine a course of action.** Jill could speak with Tim before deciding what to

do, though this may exacerbate some of his angst regarding his relationship with his sister. If she attends the wedding without consulting Tim first, this would likely cause him some amount of discomfort. However, if Jill decides not to attend the wedding and simply sends a gift, she avoids the entire debacle altogether (albeit at the expense of missing a wedding she would have liked to attend).

6. **Evaluate the selected course of action.** The best course of action is consultation first. Jill should consult with a counselor in a neighboring district who could help process different solutions and serve as a professional precaution. However, it seems that it would cause the least amount of harm to all involved if Jill simply opted not to attend.
7. **Implement the course of action.** If she does decide not to attend, Jill will have to take care to explore her emotional response to this decision in her ongoing work with Tim. It would be important to ensure that she does not harbor resentment toward him for missing the wedding or to work in supervision to manage these emotions if she does.

The Likely Answer

While it would be nice to see Marney again, the risk of harm to Tim seems to make attending the wedding the less desirable solution.

IN-CLASS DISCUSSION AND EXERCISES

Group Discussion: Theoretical Orientation

Guidelines for the counseling relationship are obviously informed by the ACA Code of Ethics, but a counselor's theoretical orientation is an important *playbook* for how the therapeutic relationship is to be managed. Some theories support closeness and personal disclosure (e.g., existential psychotherapy), whereas others support greater boundaries (e.g., cognitive therapy).

As a group, discuss your respective approaches to counseling and the theories that inform it. What will be some of the potential tripping points related to ethically managing relationships with clients? What might you need to consider in balancing the needs of your client(s), the specifics of your counseling approach, the ethics of the profession, and your own needs regarding personal disclosures and/or personal boundaries with clients?

Group Discussion: Maintaining Boundaries

Counseling is a humanistic profession, and efforts to maintain boundaries can at times require clinicians to negate the needs of their clients in favor of adherence to the code of ethics. Accepting gifts, phone calls outside of normal business hours, and even disclosure of personal information may be seen as boundary violations in some cases.

With regard to boundaries, what might be some of your areas of potential difficulty? If a client attempts to give an extravagant gift, calls repeatedly outside of scheduled appointments, or repeatedly asks you for personal information, how will you respond in a way that maintains the restrictions of the counseling relationship yet does not damage rapport? Are there certain boundaries that you anticipate will be more challenging to maintain?

Role Play: Whoops! Wrong Room

Using the scenario described in *Whoops! Wrong Room*, role-play possible outcomes. Have one member play the role of G.G. and another play the role of Mildred discussing the situation afterward. If you were Mildred, how might you actually express your sympathy and concern for what happened? As G.G., how quick would you be to forgive, and how might you respond to Mildred's apology?

Documentation: Problem, Data, Assessment, and Plan

Using the Problem, Data, Assessment, and Plan (PDAP) format, pick one of the cases and write a progress note indicating the following:

Problem: What were the presenting concerns of this particular interaction?

Data: What, objectively, has happened? Remember to write this without subjective language or interpretation.

Assessment: As the counselor or supervisor in question, what *should* be done? Be sure to demonstrate comprehensive use of the decision-making model in this section.

Plan: What *will* be done? Be sure to outline a comprehensive plan that relates to the decision-making model.

References

American School Counselor Association. (2016). *Ethical standards for school counselors.* Alexandria, VA: Author.

Baum, R. (2010). How to decline Facebook friends without offence. *Reuters.* Retrieved from https://www.reuters.com/article/us-etiquette-facebook/how-to-decline-facebook-friends-withoutoffence-idUSTRE61L1WL20100222

Bryn Athyn College. (2019). *Student handbook.* Retrieved from https://brynathyn.edu/wp-content/uploads/2016/02/UndergraduateStudentHandbook.pdf

Forester-Miller, H., & Davis, T. E. (2016). *Practitioner's guide to ethical decision-making* (Rev. ed.). Retrieved from https://www.counseling.org/docs/default-source/ethics/practioner-39-s-guide-to-ethical-decision-making.pdf?sfvrsn=10

Herlihy, B. J., Hermann, M. A., & Greden, L. R. (2014). Legal and ethical implications of using religious beliefs as the basis for refusing to counsel certain clients. *Journal of Counseling and Development,* 92(2), 148–153. doi:10.1002/j.1556-6676.2014.00142.x

Jahnke, S., Philipp, K., & Hoyer, J. (2015). Stigmatizing attitudes towards people with pedophilia and their malleability among psychotherapists in training. *Child Abuse and Neglect, 40*, 93–102. doi:10.1016/j.chiabu.2014.07.008

Lösel, F., & Schmucker, M. (2005). The effectiveness of treatment for sexual offenders: A comprehensive meta-analysis. *Journal of Experimental Criminology, 1*(1), 117–146. doi:10.1007/s11292-004-6466-7

Wampold, B. E. (2012). Humanism as a common factor in psychotherapy. *Psychotherapy, 49*, 445–449. doi:10.1037/a0027113

CHAPTER 2

CONFIDENTIALITY AND PRIVACY (SECTION B OF THE ACA CODE OF ETHICS)

INTRODUCTION

Confidentiality is critical in counseling. The public's trust in the profession to keep what is discussed with their counselor private is in many ways the cornerstone of the profession. This section provides examples of how this value—which is integral to the survival of counseling as a vocation and to the well-being of clients—can be one of the most regularly challenged ethical constructs.

All cases will be assessed using Cottone's (2001) social constructivism model for making an ethical decision.

COTTONE'S SOCIAL CONSTRUCTIVISM MODEL

While other models emphasize a linear, intrapsychic, counselor-focused approach to ethical decision-making (e.g., Forester-Miller & Davis, 2016), Cottone's social constructivism model posits a more interpersonal approach. It takes the activity out of the individual and constructs the activity as more relational, asserting that a decision is always made in interaction with at least one other individual (Cottone, 2001). In short, while efforts are made in this chapter's case examples to delineate a specific sequence of decision-making, this model is less about a set of steps and more about a consideration of processes.

Cottone suggests that when an ethical dilemma is identified, a counselor should start by acquiring relevant information from the stakeholders involved in the situation, followed by a consideration of the nature of the relationships between the stakeholders. Do those individuals have conflicting interests in terms of the outcome of the situation, or are they essentially aligned? The counselor would then consult with colleagues and the ACA Code of Ethics before beginning the more interactive processes of negotiating, working toward consensus, and reflecting interactively with further arbitration as a final step if necessary. The underlying belief is that there is no one absolute truth or singular decision that is correct for a particular dilemma; rather, the belief is that the truth is solely applicable within a particular context, as it is constructed by all of the stakeholders involved.

CONFIDENTIALITY IN COUPLES COUNSELING (*IN THE WINK OF AN EYE*)

Carl is a counselor working for a group practice in a metropolitan area. As he received a postgraduate certificate in couples counseling, he regularly treats couples for a variety of relationship concerns. His training in conflict resolution has helped him carve out a niche as the "go to clinician" for couples struggling in the aftermath of infidelity.

Carl meets with a married couple in their 30s—David and Valerie—for an intake session. As part of his systemic focus, he chooses not to meet with couples independent of one another unless there is concern of interpersonal violence. In Carl's own words posted to his public website, "I choose not to be a secret keeper for individual members of a couple … anything we do is done with everyone present." As such, his introductory session includes both partners, and his intention is usually to proceed this way for every session onward.

Once formal introductions have been made, Carl asks his standard opening question: "What brings you both here today?"

With almost no pause, Valerie is the first to respond. "I'll tell you why we're here!" she nearly shouts, her voice shaking as she looks back and forth between her husband and Carl. "This man is a liar, and he has been cheating on me for years. I can't prove it, but I know he is!"

Before Carl can even respond, she puts her head down and begins to cry. The session pushes ahead as David quickly responds. "Doc," he says, folding his arms and leaning back in his chair, "I have no idea what she's talking about. I am not cheating on her. I never have, and I never will."

What happens next is fast, but it is impossible for Carl to miss: While Valerie has her head down and is crying, David makes eye contact with Carl. Without Valerie noticing, David smiles slyly … and winks.

Questions for Discussion

1. *Regarding confidentiality, what is Carl's obligation? Who is his client?*
2. *Assuming Carl decides to confront David about the wink, how will he do so?*
3. *Assuming Carl decides to* not *confront David, how will he move forward with counseling? Does his knowing that David may have slyly admitted infidelity change his approach in any way?*

Straight From the Code

1. **B.1.b. Respect for Privacy.** Counselors respect the privacy of prospective and current clients. Counselors request private information from clients only when it is beneficial to the counseling process.
2. **B.1.c. Respect for Confidentiality.** Counselors protect the confidential information of prospective and current clients. Counselors disclose

information only with appropriate consent or with sound legal or ethical justification.

3. **B.4.b. Couples and Family Counseling.** In the absence of an agreement to the contrary, the couple or family is considered to be the client.

Applying a Decision-Making Model: Cottone's Social Constructivism Model

1. **Obtain information from those involved.** So far, Carl is aware that Valerie has suspicions of infidelity on David's behalf, but he is unclear as to the rationale for these suspicions (or David's wink, really). Carl could certainly opt to follow up by asking more about Valerie's misgivings, but this would require him to ignore the wink. If he attempts to question David regarding the reasoning behind the wink (e.g., Was it an effort to assure him that he was not cheating? Was he trying to clandestinely admit to having an affair as a way to make a connection with the counselor without Valerie knowing?), he risks damaging rapport irreparably.

   Obtaining additional information at this time seems less than plausible, and Carl is in something of a *no-win* scenario: If he acknowledges the wink, he risks losing rapport with David, which is critical to any success he hopes to obtain moving forward. If he opts to ignore it, he is potentially betraying Valerie's trust.

2. **Assess the nature of the relationships operating at that moment in time.** Carl has clearly identified himself as a couples counselor, though he may lack some clarity regarding how this affects his treatment of individuals *within* a couple. Is he still beholden to the rules of confidentiality as they apply to David and Valerie as individuals, or does he eschew these needs in favor of the "greater good"?

3. **Consult with colleagues or the ACA Code of Ethics.** Carl does not have time to consult with a colleague or the code before he responds in the moment, so his only hope is to have a working understanding of the ACA Code of Ethics.

   The concern at hand is one of fidelity. Specifically, who is Carl's client, and what does it mean to abide by the rules of confidentiality in this scenario? In consulting the code, one of the first problems noted is a discrepancy between subsections B.1.b. and B.1.c. Based on the wording in B.1.b., which states, "Counselors request private information from clients only when it is beneficial to the counseling process," Carl would be correct in assuming it is appropriate to ask David why he winked. He could argue that this was the best course of action as (a) the "information" was not private, in that it was disclosed in session with the other partner present (even if she did not see it), and

(b) the "information" disclosed is beneficial to the counseling process, given that *not* acknowledging it negates a significant interpersonal process.

However, based on the wording in B.1.c., which states, "Counselors disclose information only with appropriate consent," Carl would also be correct in assuming it is *inappropriate* to ask David why he winked. He could argue that this was the best course of action as the "information" was clearly disclosed without wanting David's partner to know. As David is a part of his client (the couple), he is obligated to provide him confidentiality, and it seems clear from the subtlety of the interaction that this is *not* something David wants shared with his wife.

4. **Negotiate when there is a disagreement.** Though the case does not indicate if Carl managed to get the couple to sign a consent form as well as an explanation of services, it certainly highlights the importance of signing all relevant intake paperwork before beginning counseling. However, even if the paperwork has not yet been signed, section B.4.b. states, "In the absence of an agreement to the contrary, the couple or family is considered to be the client." As such, we can discern that the couple is Carl's client, and decision-making moving forward should likely put couple-related concerns first.

5. **Respond in a way that allows for reasonable consensus regarding next steps.** While opting not to acknowledge this interaction in the interest of maintaining rapport with David is a viable option, Carl discussing the wink in session may be the better decision. The couple is his client, and this information affects all parties moving forward. His decision to not disclose this interaction could rightly be seen by Valerie as complicit should it come to light in the future. Cottone (2001) has also indicated the importance of awareness of constructivist factors that affect the decision-making process, and there are significant contextual variables at play here: Carl is a male clinician, and David is the male partner, which puts Valerie in a potentially uncomfortable position as the only female in this dynamic.

   Nevertheless, this would require some introspection regarding concerns and motivations. It is important for clinicians to be aware of potential *bias hot spots* (Jacob, Roth, Cliento, & Stoler, 2015) and the impact this can have on the counseling process. Specifically, does Carl have personal biases related to infidelity that motivate this decision? Is there something about David's presentation—his sly demeanor, his clear disregard for his wife's trust—that evokes an emotional response from Carl? If Carl decides to discuss the wink with the couple, he will need to carefully monitor his emotional response in the moment as well as afterward. For example, if he finds that he enjoys exposing David to his wife by pointedly asking, "Did you just wink at me?" this is useful content for a discussion with his supervisor.

The Likely Answer

Discussing the wink in session may be the best choice.

CONFIDENTIALITY IN PUBLIC SETTINGS (*FEELING EXPOSED*)

Devon is a counselor in private practice in a rural area. The town he lives in is about 200 miles from any major metropolitan areas, and the total population is under 20,000. It is not the smallest town in the world, but Devon has run into a few of his clients in the community and is careful to mention the possibility of chance encounters with clients upon intake.

Devon is a health enthusiast and attends a local gym 3 or 4 days a week—"The only decent one in town," according to him. Upon finishing his workout one day, he showers, puts on a towel, begins to walk to his locker ... and notices that three of his clients are standing in the locker room in various states of undress. These clients do not know each other—one he sees for couples counseling, and the other two he sees individually—and are currently unaware that Devon is standing just a few feet away. They all just happen to attend the same gym, and they all just happen to be in the same exact spot.

Thankfully, Devon remembers having explained the basics of confidentiality with all of these clients during intake, even going so far as to make them aware that chance encounters in the community might be possible. His standard overview has typically been to let clients know that if he sees them in public, he will not acknowledge their presence unless they approach him first.

At first glance, none of the clients seem aware of Devon's presence ... but he really needs to get dressed and head to work.

Questions for Discussion

1. *Regarding confidentiality, what is Devon's obligation to his clients?*
2. *Regarding privacy, what is Devon's obligation to himself in this moment?*
3. *How will Devon manage this concern with his clients moving forward?*

Straight From the Code

1. **B.1.b. Respect for Privacy.** Counselors respect the privacy of prospective and current clients. Counselors request private information from clients only when it is beneficial to the counseling process.

2. **B.1.c. Respect for Confidentiality.** Counselors protect the confidential information of prospective and current clients. Counselors disclose information only with appropriate consent or with sound legal or ethical justification.

3. **B.1.d. Explanation of Limitations.** At initiation and throughout the counseling process, counselors inform clients of the limitations of confidentiality and seek to identify situations in which confidentiality must be breached.

Applying a Decision-Making Model: Cottone's Social Constructivism Model

1. **Obtain information from those involved.** In this case, any information obtained would have to come from contextual information that can be gleaned from the moment (e.g., to what extent do these individuals seem to be either aware of Devon's presence or uncomfortable with the current situation?) or previous information obtained from past sessions (e.g., have any of these individuals previously provided information in session or otherwise that would indicate a situation such as this could be upsetting?).

2. **Assess the nature of the relationships operating at that moment in time.** Devon is a counselor for all three of these individuals, but he is not acting as their counselor in this moment. Regardless, he is still bound by the ethics of his profession.

3. **Consult with colleagues or the ACA Code of Ethics.** In short, consulting is not an option in this moment. It is to be hoped that Devon is aware of the Code's basics and will document his decision-making process as soon as he is able to.

   Based on the wording in B.1.b., which states, "Counselors respect the privacy of prospective and current clients," as well as his discussion of protocol for chance meetings in public, Devon is likely correct in his decision to not approach any of these clients. However, the Code does not explicitly outline how to manage seeing clients in a public setting, and the extent to which the counselor's own comfort level with these interactions factors into decision-making. It is not clear to what extent it is appropriate to engage (or *not* engage) any of them if they reach out to him directly, or if he is entitled to privacy if he feels uncomfortable with their efforts at communication.

   This wording in B.1.c. does not provide much in the way of additional guidance, but it does highlight that confidentiality operates in two directions: Counselors should not divulge *or* request information from clients without their consent. In this moment, it is important that Devon makes every effort to refrain both from indicating publicly that any of these three individuals are his clients and from engaging in any conversation *not* connected to counseling that might accidentally reveal confidential information. If he does interact with any of them in any way, he should avoid asking questions or saying anything that might identify these individuals as clients publicly.

As previously stated, Devon has explained the basics of confidentiality with his clients, though the wording in B.1.d. also explicitly states that explanations should continue "throughout the counseling process" as well. This would suggest that Devon should make an effort to discuss this incident during the next counseling meeting with each of these individuals, and negotiation will have to occur regarding how the gym will be managed moving forward. Are these three individuals uncomfortable with the idea that Devon attends the same health club? Are there ways to negotiate when Devon attends the facility to reduce the likelihood of an encounter? Is there a balance that can be established regarding the needs of these clients *and* Devon?

4. **Negotiate when there is a disagreement.** The code does not state that Devon should quit the club or refuse to do so if any of the individuals requests it, but it would require negotiation. If Devon is uncomfortable being approached in public settings—locker rooms in particular—he should make clients aware of this if an encounter like this might happen again.

5. **Respond in a way that allows for reasonable consensus regarding next steps.** In the moment, Devon needs to *read the room* and make his best effort to respond in a way that meets the needs of all parties involved. If none of the clients acknowledge him or make obvious efforts to avoid acknowledgment, he needs to respond in kind. If they do approach him in a way that makes him uncomfortable or creates concerns regarding his own needs for appropriate boundaries, he will have to address this in the moment or in a subsequent counseling session. During the next sessions with all three clients, he should discuss the incident with them and make an effort to negotiate compromises moving forward that would best address the needs and concerns of all involved.

   However, Devon should also consider the possibility that if any of these individuals indicate they are comfortable with the possibility of continued contact, they may be responding politely instead of genuinely. Devon needs to be certain that he maintains a connection with his clients that promotes honesty. In a situation like this, it is easy to imagine a client feigning politeness despite personal discomfort, perhaps in favor of avoiding a complicated conversation.

The Likely Answer

Devon needs to take a deep breath, get dressed, and then talk it over with everyone during the next counseling session.

CONFIDENTIALITY IN PUBLIC SETTINGS CONTINUED (*BABY, YOU CAN DRIVE MY CAR ... OR CAN YOU?*)

Howard is a counselor working for a drug and alcohol counseling program in a metropolitan area, and he is currently seeing a great deal of court-ordered clients for supportive treatment following convictions for drug- and alcohol-related charges. After work, Howard is scheduled to meet a few friends for dinner at a local upscale restaurant—so upscale, in fact, that it has valet parking.

Howard has agreed to act as the designated driver for this evening and arrives at the valet parking entrance with three of his friends in the car. He opens the door, reaches out to hand his keys to the valet, and immediately realizes that the valet is a current client: Varg, a young man he has been seeing for individual counseling for 3 months.

Varg immediately looks uncomfortable and does not acknowledge his connection to Howard but instead continues to extend his hand, waiting for the keys. Howard is aware of Varg's recent criminal past, namely a conviction for identity theft to support an opiate dependency. He is also aware that Varg failed his last urine screen, testing positive for both opiates and cocaine.

To make matters worse, Howard cannot exactly remember, but he thinks his passport might be in his car's glove compartment.

Questions for Discussion

1. *Regarding confidentiality, what is Howard's obligation to his client?*
2. *Regarding his own sense of security and well-being, what is Howard's obligation to himself in this moment?*
3. *Whatever Howard decides to do in this moment, how will he discuss this with Varg during their next meeting?*

Straight From the Code

1. **B.1.b. Respect for Privacy.** Counselors respect the privacy of prospective and current clients. Counselors request private information from clients only when it is beneficial to the counseling process.

2. **B.1.c. Respect for Confidentiality.** Counselors protect the confidential information of prospective and current clients. Counselors disclose information only with appropriate consent or with sound legal or ethical justification.

3. **B.1.d. Explanation of Limitations.** At initiation and throughout the counseling process, counselors inform clients of the limitations of confidentiality and seek to identify situations in which confidentiality must be breached.

Applying a Decision-Making Model: Cottone's Social Constructivism Model

1. **Obtain information from those involved.** In this case, time is of the essence, and the ability to gain insight from contextual information is compromised. Howard is literally about to hand his keys to the valet; an extended pause to carefully decide whether or not he should drive away and park somewhere else would elicit suspicion from his friends and may make for some great discomfort on Varg's end as well. If Howard's friends are aware of his vocation, knowing that Varg is a client would likely disclose to the group that this individual is in counseling, struggles with a drug dependency, and was recently arrested.

2. **Assess the nature of the relationships operating at that moment in time.** As in the previous case example, Howard is Varg's counselor, but he is not acting as his counselor in this moment. Regardless, he is still bound by the ethics of his profession. Additionally, Varg is now filling the role of service provider to Howard, in that he is being paid to care for Howard's car, and Howard may be expected to provide him with a tip once services are rendered.

3. **Consult with colleagues or the ACA Code of Ethics.** Also similar to the previous case example, this is not an option in this moment. It is once again to be hoped that Howard is aware of the Code's basic policies and will document his decision-making process as soon as he is able.

   Based on B.1.b., we can likely deduce that Howard should take all measures to make sure he does not "out" Varg as a client to any of his friends. He needs to be aware that disclosing confidential information is not limited just to a direct admission to his friends that Varg is a client in therapy—as stated, a hesitation in the moment could disclose just as much.

   Again, the wording in B.1.c. does not provide much in the way of additional guidance, but it highlights once more that confidentiality operates in two directions: Counselors should not divulge *or* request information from clients without their consent. Howard must not indicate to anyone that Varg is his client, but he also must refrain from engaging in any conversation *not* connected to counseling that might accidentally reveal confidential information. Specifically, he should avoid both asking questions and saying anything that might identify Varg as a client to either Howard's friends or Varg's employers and coworkers.

   The example does not explicitly state so, but it is expected that Howard has explained the basics of confidentiality to Varg during intake. The wording in B.1.d. also states that explanations should continue "throughout the counseling process" as well, and Howard should make an effort to discuss this incident during the next counseling meeting with Varg regardless of his decision in the moment. If it is in any way likely that Howard and Varg will regularly see each other in public, how these moments are to be handled moving forward should be carefully negotiated.

4. **Negotiate when there is a disagreement.** The Code does not explicitly state that Howard must hand over his keys or that he has the right to refuse to engage in services with a client that involve having the client drive his car. However, if Howard gives over his keys, this situation creates a dual relationship that is unavoidable in this moment: Varg will be both his client *and* his valet. If Howard opts not to hand over the keys and chooses another option regarding parking, he risks offending the client and/or indirectly violating his confidentiality.

   An additional concern is the conflict between Varg's need for confidentiality and Howard's need for personal safety (particularly as his passport might be accessible to the client). However, it is important to recognize that encounters with individuals with criminal records in positions of service are common occurrences. In the United States, it is estimated that close to one in 10 citizens has a felony conviction (Shannon et al., 2017), and the Substance Abuse and Mental Health Services Administration estimates the same number struggle with drug abuse (National Institute on Drug Abuse, 2015). Howard is simply aware of the risk in this moment, but encounters such as this are likely a daily occurrence for most individuals who interact with the public regularly in any way.

5. **Respond in a way that allows for reasonable consensus regarding next steps.** Howard has every right to refuse to hand over his keys and drive to another lot for parking; he could even make up a story to his friends about needing to save money by finding a cheaper lot. However, this will at the very least cause damage to the therapeutic relationship (though Varg might prefer not to have engaged in this interaction as well) and may unintentionally violate confidentiality. If Howard is trying to protect himself from harm, it would serve to reason that Varg would be unlikely to risk violating an individual who is aware of his criminal record.

The Likely Answer

Howard should smile, hand over the keys, check the glove compartment and grab his passport if it is there, and tip the standard 15% once he gets his car back.

THIRD-PARTY REQUESTS FOR INFORMATION (*IN THE CRIMINAL JUSTICE SYSTEM…*)

Mariska works as a counselor in a methadone maintenance program in an urban setting. Clients are individuals struggling with opiate dependency receiving medication-assisted treatment (methadone) to address physical symptoms of withdrawal. Mariska has been at the clinic for just under a year now, but she is well aware of the social stigma that most of her clients attach to methadone treatment. Many indicate not telling their friends or family members about this treatment for fear of judgment, and the clinic directors regularly highlight the importance of confidentiality in staff meetings.

Belzer is a new client of Mariska's and has just attended an initial intake session. During this initial meeting, he indicated that he is facing an upcoming court date for a possession charge and might need a record of treatment attendance, but he does not say much else about the matter. The intake takes place on a Thursday, and a follow-up meeting is scheduled for Monday.

On Friday, Mariska receives a phone call from an individual claiming to be Belzer's attorney. The attorney says that he is representing Belzer, who is facing jail time for a robbery. The attorney asks Mariska to forward a letter indicating that Belzer attended an intake session and is willing to attend drug treatment. Mariska states that she does not have a release signed to provide this information, and the attorney responds by saying that Belzer will likely go to jail if she does not fax or email verification of treatment attendance within the hour and that Belzer cannot leave court to sign a form.

Questions for Discussion

1. *Regarding confidentiality, what is Mariska's obligation to Belzer?*
2. *Is there a way to gain consent without having Belzer come back to the office to sign a release?*
   a. *Are consents obtained over the phone or through video conferencing valid?*

Straight From the Code

1. **B.1.c. Respect for Confidentiality.** Counselors protect the confidential information of prospective and current clients. Counselors disclose information only with appropriate consent or with sound legal or ethical justification.

2. **B.1.d. Explanation of Limitations.** At initiation and throughout the counseling process, counselors inform clients of the limitations of confidentiality and seek to identify situations in which confidentiality must be breached.

3. **B.2.a. Serious and Foreseeable Harm and Legal Requirements.** The general requirement that counselors keep information confidential does not apply when disclosure is required to protect clients or identified others from serious and foreseeable harm or when legal requirements demand that confidential information must be revealed. Counselors consult with other professionals when in doubt as to

the validity of an exception. Additional considerations apply when addressing end-of-life issues.

4. **B.3.e. Transmitting Confidential Information.** Counselors take precautions to ensure the confidentiality of all information transmitted through the use of any medium.

Applying a Decision-Making Model: Cottone's Social Constructivism Model

1. **Obtain information from those involved.** To release information to a third party, counselors must have the client sign a release form that clearly outlines the parameters of information to be released and is signed directly by the client. One of Mariska's main problems is that there is no way to verify that Belzer is willing to have this information released to the court without using video conferencing or the telephone. Some clinicians may opt to use fax or email to obtain consent, and email portals are becoming increasingly common for client paperwork. However, this does not provide any guarantee that the individual signing is indeed who they say they are.

2. **Assess the nature of the relationships operating at that moment in time.** Though she has only met him for one session, Mariska is without a doubt Belzer's counselor and is obligated to provide services in accordance with the ACA Code of Ethics. An intake session occurred, and the specifics of this relationship (Mariska as the counselor and Belzer as the client) have been established.

3. **Consult with colleagues or the ACA Code of Ethics.** Mariska should definitely pause to review the Code and to discuss the matter with a direct supervisor. Her supervisor or agency of employment may have specific standards regarding release of information, but her ultimate concern is providing services in accordance with the ethics of her profession.

   In all cases, clients' confidentiality is critical. The nature of this specific treatment carries significant stigma, with many methadone maintenance patients indicating concerns about the negative public perception of methadone treatment and its perceived consequences (Woo et al., 2017). As such, no information should be released to any party unless it is absolutely clear that the client condones it. Still, it is unlikely that the attorney is anyone other than who he claims to be, and Mariska has a responsibility to her client to ensure that his requests are verified and honored.

   As part of the intake process, Mariska should have provided Belzer with a clear overview of treatment specifics, and explanations of confidentiality should have been included in the consent to treatment. Explanation of treatment details (confidentiality, payment, etc.) should have been discussed and verified by client signature during the intake session.

It is important to note that a possibility of incarceration does not constitute protection from serious and foreseeable harm. Also, *legal requirements* (B.2.a.) likely refer to something along the lines of a court order, which is different from a request issued by an attorney. In the case of a court order, counselors are obligated to provide the information requested or face legal consequences for not doing so. In the case of a request for information, counselors are obligated to respond, but not necessarily to divulge all information requested. However, Mariska should do what she can to act in the best interest of her client, and keeping him out of jail is likely what he would prefer. As such, she should try to see if there is a way to release the information required without violating the Code or the law.

Per the wording in B.3.e., counselors have to make sure that the information requested by a third party—if she chooses to send it—is handled with the utmost care. Unfortunately, emails and faxes require a network of computers to transmit this information, and ensuring absolute confidence is almost impossible. While there is no specific wording in the Code that forbids the use of email or fax to obtain consent to release information, the counselor would need to be sure that the limitations of this means of transmission are clearly outlined. The release of information should likely indicate that the client agrees to have this information faxed or emailed and is aware of the risks inherent in doing so.

4. **Negotiate when there is a disagreement.** A disagreement does not appear to be evident. The Code states that counselors maintain the confidence of the client but that they can obtain consent to have this information released.

5. **Respond in a way that allows for reasonable consensus regarding next steps.** Mariska may have the option to send Belzer a release of information via fax or email, have him sign it with a witness present, and then fax or email it back to her. She could then release the information requested, also via fax or email. However, the release should make mention of the limitations of confidentiality via electronic means. Electronic communications are—in theory—treated the same as any other client–counselor communication in that confidentiality abides with certain exceptions (e.g., suicidal threats, supervision). The concern is that email, texts, faxes, and voice mail cannot be afforded the same guarantees of confidentiality as face-to-face contact in session due to the lack of security measures beyond simply password protecting an email account.

The Likely Answer

Mariska can probably take care of this through fax or email, though she might want to be more careful to get releases signed in advance if the client says anything about a court appearance requiring a record of attendance.

CONFIDENTIALITY RELATED TO CONTAGIOUS OR LIFE-THREATENING DISEASES (*A LOSE–LOSE SITUATION*)

Patricia is a counselor in a community-based setting that deals predominantly with drug and alcohol treatment. She has been seeing Jason—a 26-year-old male struggling with opiate addiction—for approximately 6 months. Counseling overall has been going well, and Patricia reports feeling that there is a connection between her and Jason. Content of counseling has focused mostly on insight and development of sober coping skills.

For today's session, Jason is excited to discuss a new relationship. He reports that he has been dating Angela for about 2 weeks now and that he is "ridiculously happy." He says that it is likely too early to tell but that he is "almost definitely falling in love with her."

After listening to further descriptions of Angela and her background, Patricia realizes that Angela—a 36-year-old female also struggling with opiate addiction—is a client in one of her groups at the same community-based clinic. Patricia is aware that Angela has hepatitis C. Based on the content of counseling with Jason, she believes that Jason is unaware of Angela's diagnosis.

In short, the counselor in this case knows that Jason is romantically involved with another client who has a potentially communicable disease (hepatitis C), but Jason is unaware of the diagnosis.

Questions for Discussion

1. *Regarding protection from harm, what is Patricia's obligation to Jason?*
2. *Regarding confidentiality, what is Patricia's obligation to Jason?*
3. *Regarding confidentiality, what is Patricia's obligation to Angela?*

Straight From the Code

1. **B.1.c. Respect for Confidentiality.** Counselors protect the confidential information of prospective and current clients. Counselors disclose information only with appropriate consent or with sound legal or ethical justification.

2. **B.1.d. Explanation of Limitations.** At initiation and throughout the counseling process, counselors inform clients of the limitations of confidentiality and seek to identify situations in which confidentiality must be breached.

3. **B.2.a. Serious and Foreseeable Harm and Legal Requirements.** The general requirement that counselors keep information confidential does not apply when disclosure is required to protect clients or identified others from serious and foreseeable harm or when legal requirements demand that confidential information must be revealed. Counselors consult with other professionals when in doubt as to the validity of an exception. Additional considerations apply when addressing end-of-life issues.

4. **B.2.c. Contagious, Life-Threatening Diseases.** When clients disclose that they have a disease commonly known to be both communicable and life-threatening, counselors may be justified in disclosing information to identifiable third parties, if the parties are known to be at serious and foreseeable risk of contracting the disease. Prior to making a disclosure, counselors assess the intent of clients to inform the third parties about their disease or to engage in any behaviors that may be harmful to an identifiable third party. Counselors adhere to relevant state laws concerning disclosure about disease status.

Applying a Decision-Making Model: Cottone's Social Constructivism Model

1. **Obtain information from those involved.** As Patricia sees Angela in a group setting and has had no indication of the relationship from Angela's perspective, she is limited to whatever information she can obtain from Jason. It will be important to ask Jason about specific risk-taking behaviors he is engaging in. For example, is he refraining from IV drug use? If he is engaging in IV drug use, does he share needles? Patricia could ask about any number of risk-taking behaviors, but it will be important to refrain from accidentally revealing specific concerns that would lead Jason to conclude that Patricia knows Angela in some way.

2. **Assess the nature of the relationships operating at that moment in time.** Though she only sees her for group, Patricia is indeed a counselor for Angela and is obligated to maintain her confidentiality. A concerning factor is that Patricia is also Jason's counselor, and she is obligated to protect him from foreseeable harm.

3. **Consult with colleagues or the ACA Code of Ethics.** An important step in this process is consulting with someone in the medical profession who is aware of the risks of transmission and the outcomes of treatment regarding hepatitis C. Per the Centers for Disease Control and Prevention (CDC), sexual contact makes it less likely for transmission of the disease to occur, though IV drug use—particularly sharing needles with another person infected with the disease—increases the risk substantially (CDC, 2019). The CDC also states that newer treatments of hepatitis C are in many cases capable of eradicating the

disease completely. Regardless of what she can determine from the CDC's website, Patricia should likely consult (and document the consultation) with a medical professional regarding the likelihood of risk.

In all cases, the clients' confidentiality is critical. Patricia should ideally find a way to maintain the confidentiality of both clients, though balancing this with concerns for Jason's safety may require her not to make the *correct* decision, but the decision that will cause the least harm.

As part of the intake process, Patricia should have provided both Jason and Angela with a clear overview of treatment specifics, and explanations of confidentiality should have been included in the consent to treatment. Explanation of treatment details (confidentiality, payment, etc.) should be discussed and verified by client signature during the intake session, regardless of whether the treatment will take place in an individual or group setting.

However, the confusing aspect of section B.2.a. (as it applies to this case) is the definition of serious and foreseeable harm. Patricia will have to determine if a possible exposure to hepatitis C meets this criterion.

Again, the wording in B.2.c. is *serious and foreseeable*, and Patricia will have to make a decision—based on information obtained from Jason regarding risk-taking behaviors as well as consultation with medical professionals—whether Jason is in imminent danger.

4. **Negotiate when there is a disagreement.** If Patricia does not tell Jason what she knows, he could contract hepatitis C and risk further complications from the illness. However, the evidence suggests that rates of contraction are low and that the disease would be easily treated (unless Jason is infected and unaware). If she tells Jason what she knows about Angela, she is without question violating her confidentiality, with regard to both a medical condition and her status as a client receiving psychotherapy.

5. **Respond in a way that allows for reasonable consensus regarding next steps.** If Jason is unaware that his partner is infected and becomes infected himself, it could potentially create a lifetime of problems and related health concerns. He would likely be culpable for this outcome to a great extent, as the risk-taking behaviors of needle sharing and unprotected sex are potentially dangerous no matter what the circumstances. If Patricia opts to explain what she knows to Jason, she is solely responsible for the impact this has on Angela.

The Likely Answer

Patricia should remind Jason of the importance of safe sex if the conversation comes up, and she should do her best to not acknowledge to either Jason or Angela that she knows the other.

REQUEST FOR INFORMATION FROM PARENTS (*HAPPY BIRTHDAY!*)

Ágúst is a counselor in a private practice where he works predominantly with adolescents. He begins seeing Orri—a 13-year-old boy—for individual counseling. Orri's parents initiated treatment, as they were worried that Orri was struggling with depression and that he may be using drugs. Six months into treatment, Orri seems to be connecting with Ágúst and has been willing to discuss some of his struggles with depression, drugs, and alcohol abuse.

Another milestone occurs at the 6-month mark of treatment, as Orri has now turned 14. As Ágúst practices in Pennsylvania, this means that Orri is now permitted to make decisions about his own treatment. He decides to continue with counseling, as he has found having a safe space to vent his frustrations to be useful.

Shortly after his 14th birthday, Orri's mother contacts Ágúst and states that she is worried that her son is abusing prescription drugs. Ágúst informs her of the limits of confidentiality, as Orri is now of the age where he can make decisions about his own treatment and that Ágúst cannot release any information without Orri's consent.

Orris' mother asks for all of Ágúst's records before Orri turned 14.

Questions for Discussion

1. *Regarding confidentiality, what is Ágúst's obligation to Orri?*
2. *Does being 14 now affect Orri's records retrospectively?*
3. *Whether Ágúst decides to release the records or not, how will he proceed with Orri's treatment?*

Straight From the Code

1. **B.5.a. Responsibility to Clients.** When counseling minor clients or adult clients who lack the capacity to give voluntary, informed consent, counselors protect the confidentiality of information received—in any medium—in the counseling relationship as specified by federal and state laws, written policies, and applicable ethical standards.

2. **B.5.b. Responsibility to Parents and Legal Guardians.** Counselors inform parents and legal guardians about the role of counselors and the confidential nature of the counseling relationship, consistent with current legal and custodial arrangements. Counselors are sensitive to the cultural diversity of families and respect the inherent rights and responsibilities of parents/guardians regarding the welfare of their children/charges according to law. Counselors work to establish, as appropriate, collaborative relationships with parents/guardians to best serve clients.

3. **B.5.c. Release of Confidential Information.** When counseling minor clients or adult clients who lack the capacity to give voluntary consent to release confidential information, counselors seek permission from an appropriate third party to disclose information. In such instances, counselors inform clients consistent with their level of understanding and take appropriate measures to safeguard client confidentiality.

Applying a Decision-Making Model: Cottone's Social Constructivism Model

1. **Obtain information from those involved.** Ágúst should likely begin this process by first asking Orri's mother what she hopes to gain from having access to her son's records. Does she have specific concerns about Orri's safety that Ágúst is unaware of? Is she aware of Ágúst's responsibility to contact Orri's legal guardian if he believed Orri to be in some form of imminent danger? Ágúst should also consult with Orri before making a decision to release any information to see if there is another way to resolve his mother's concerns. Would he be willing to allow his mother to have access to his psychotherapy records? Would it be possible to have her attend one of Orri's individual sessions to address her concerns?

2. **Assess the nature of the relationships operating at that moment in time.** Ágúst must verify that Orri meets the criteria as a child in the state in which this is occurring. For mental health treatment, the legal age of consent ranges from 12 to 16 depending on the state (Kerwin et al., 2015), though Pennsylvania has set the age at 14. It seems that the nature of this relationship at present is clear: Ágúst is indeed Orri's individual counselor, and Orri meets the criteria necessary to make determinations about his own treatment (including disclosure of records).

3. **Consult with colleagues or the ACA Code of Ethics.** One of the problems that Ágúst faces is that the Code does not explicitly state how the records of former child clients are managed. The aforementioned sections of the code (B.5.a–c) clearly outline the limits and concerns of providing counseling to a minor client, but Orri is no longer a minor in the world of mental health treatment.

   As such, confidentiality likely applies here, as Orri's age means that he retains ownership of his records both past and present (Kerwin et al., 2015). If Ágúst worked for a clinic or agency, it would be in his best interest to consult with his supervisors to determine what protocols were in place for release of records. In this case, it might be useful (though not absolutely necessary) to consult with an attorney.

4. **Negotiate when there is a disagreement.** The disagreement here is likely between Orri and his mother, though Ágúst should be careful

regarding how he addresses Orri's mother's request. It seems unlikely that such a discrepancy would result in a lawsuit, but tone of voice alone has a storied connection to malpractice (Ambady et al., 2002). It is unlikely that Orri will allow his mother to have access to his entire record, but he might be willing to have her attend one of his individual sessions.

5. **Respond in a way that allows for reasonable consensus regarding next steps.** Ágúst probably cannot justify allowing Orri's mother access to his records, but Orri has the ultimate authority regarding what happens next. Ágúst could suggest that Orri's mother attend an individual session as a way of placating her, but Orri is not obligated to let her attend if he is uncomfortable with this.

The Likely Answer

Ágúst should tell Orri's mother, "No, I can't give you access to Orri's records, but let me talk to Orri and see if we can all meet together to discuss your concerns."

MULTICULTURAL/DIVERSITY CONSIDERATIONS (*DETERMINING WHAT THE SYSTEMIC LENS ENTAILS*)

Gabriel is a counselor in private practice in the downtown area of a large urban community. He is on numerous insurance panels and sees mostly individuals who work in the city and wish to use their private health insurance benefits. He markets himself as a practitioner who is open to and affirming of all types of diverse identities, and he prides himself on having created a space that reflects this value.

Today, Gabriel is meeting with a couple for an initial session. When he greets the couple, he is admittedly surprised because the husband is wearing a thobe, the wife is wearing a niqab, and this is the first time he will have worked with anybody of the Islamic faith. As the session progresses, the husband explains that the rules of his religion permit him to have more than one wife if he is able to financially provide for all of them. He explains that he has four wives and that the partner with him in the session is his third wife. His wife asserts that she is fine with being one of the four wives and that this is not the problem in their relationship.

Gabriel tries to maintain composure, but internally he is both confused and conflicted as he does not believe in polygamy, and he has never encountered this dynamic, either personally or professionally. His initial reaction is to feel inadequate as a professional and ill equipped to offer any meaningful support to a couple whose family culture is so profoundly different from his. He feels a bit panicked and wants to refer the couple to a colleague because he knows nothing about Muslim or Islamic culture and is uncomfortable with the idea of marital therapy involving a relationship that potentially involves more than two individuals.

Questions for Discussion

1. *Is Gabriel doing couples or family work when counseling a polygamous couple, and who should have access to the information discussed in sessions?*
2. *How will Gabriel be able to work with a couple with a framework so profoundly unfamiliar to him?*
3. *Should Gabriel refer this couple to a counselor who has experience with Muslim clients or who is Muslim themselves?*

Straight From the Code

1. **B.1.a. Multicultural/Diversity Considerations.** Counselors maintain awareness and sensitivity regarding cultural meanings of confidentiality and privacy. Counselors respect differing views toward disclosure of information. Counselors hold ongoing discussions with clients as to how, when, and with whom information is to be shared.
2. **B.4.b.** In couples and family counseling, counselors clearly define who is considered "the client" and discuss expectations and limitations of confidentiality. Counselors seek agreement and document in writing such agreement among all involved parties regarding the confidentiality of information. In the absence of an agreement to the contrary, the couple or family is considered to be the client.

Applying a Decision-Making Model: Cottone's Social Constructivism Model

1. **Obtain information from those involved.** The first step of this model applies perfectly to this particular situation because Gabriel is uninformed about the family culture of this couple, and his lack of awareness has made him feel inadequate. The Cottone model gives Gabriel permission to admit to his clients that he does not fully understand their religion and culture and to ask them to teach him about it. This begins the ethical decision-making process and makes the circumstances transparent to both Gabriel and his clients. This also suggests that future decisions regarding the issue can be more easily made, not in a vacuum but rather in the context of the relationship between Gabriel and the couple, as is called for by the model (Cottone, 2001). Gabriel should take this opportunity to be vulnerable, to acknowledge his limitations, and to enable his clients to be the experts and to teach him. This helps him to learn, to avoid judgment or imposition of his own values, and to also give power to the clients themselves. In addition, Gabriel should be prepared to educate himself more thoroughly on relevant aspects of the Islamic faith so that he can more effectively engage with this couple.

2. **Assess the nature of the relationship operating at that moment in time.** This is also an important and necessary step for Gabriel in his developing therapeutic relationship with this couple. They came to see him as a married couple; however, the larger context of the family within which they function actually involves three other women who are actively contributing to the couple's dynamic. Gabriel will need to discuss matters of clinical work and confidentiality with the couple in the room with him. In addition, together and collaboratively, they will need to come to a clear definition of the couple and of the client and determine who will be discussed and who ultimately has access to information about the work. The clients themselves will have to work with Gabriel to clarify if the work being done is considered couples work and is just between the two of them, marital therapy that involves the other wives, or family therapy. These boundaries will need to be discussed and negotiated, and Gabriel will have to resign himself to the fact that the nature and the relationship he will have with this couple may be different than the relationships he has had with other client couples. He may even find that he and the clients are at odds and in conflict with the way they perceive the relationship. However, according to the Cottone model, the structure of the relationship they construct together, through negotiation, consensualizing, and arbitration, if necessary, will be appropriate to the social consensual domain within which they will interact. The social constructivist approach to ethical decision-making "define[s] the view within a social consensual domain as *absolutely true* within that social context" (Cottone, 2001). What works with this couple will be distinct and may not be appropriate in any other therapeutic relationship, and the model allows for and encourages this. Gabriel and this couple will also need to discuss the extent to which they need or desire their Islamic faith to be a part of their therapeutic work.

3. **Consult with colleagues or the ACA Code of Ethics.** Best practice would likely encourage Gabriel to do both of these steps, gaining an understanding of the standard expected as articulated in the ACA Code, while also seeking the expert opinions of counselors with practical experience. B.1.a. indicates that a counselor should maintain ongoing discussions with clients regarding with whom information about the work should be disclosed. This reinforces the collaborative and consensual approach that is advanced by the Cottone model. B.4.b. does the same in encouraging a clear definition of who the client is and the boundaries of confidentiality, going so far as to encourage the counselor to get that definition in writing so there can be no doubt. Through discussion, the client is actively involved in this process as well. Gabriel should also consult with another counselor. He should do this not only to gain insight from someone who may have had experience working with Muslim clients, but also so that he can be

honest and clear about his values regarding polygamy to ensure that it does not interfere with his ability to do solid work with this couple. After having consulted another counselor, Gabriel should only refer the clients if he determines that he is unable to bracket his own values enough to be ethical and effective. If he can do so, with consultation and support, to refer them would be unethical and discriminatory.

4. **Negotiate when there is a disagreement.** This step is in place because counselors and clients may feel differently about various aspects of the therapeutic relationship and the work that is being done within it. Gabriel and his clients may have differing opinions about with whom clinical information should be shared, both in the beginning and later on in their relationship. In the case of this type of disagreement, the process of negotiation and arbitration, if ultimately necessary, are available to the counselor and clients. The hope is that the negotiation and consensualizing processes would render arbitration unnecessary, as it may have unintended but clinically significant consequences on the relationship. Gabriel will need to be willing to give his clients enough voice and freedom to express genuine disagreement with him but still remain aligned with them in the relationship.

5. **Respond in a way that allows for reasonable consensus regarding next steps.** At this point, Gabriel and his clients would have come to a relatively clear decision about who the clients are, who has access to clinical information, and how to proceed with the relationship. If a point of disagreement arises, the model advises that Gabriel should go back to the process of negotiation and consensualizing as necessary. The model also encourages "interactive reflection" or "a period of reflection and active processing of what the counselor intends to do" (Tarvydas, 1998). As indicated by the name, this process should be contextual and social, rather than intrapsychic in nature, and both expert opinions and the client's concerns should be considered.

The Likely Answer

This process of defining the "couple" should be done within the context of the clinical relationship, the distinct nature of the clients' marriage, and their faith. Gabriel should learn from the clients, in addition to doing his own research, about this specific type of Islamic marriage. Gabriel should not refer these clients to another practitioner unless, after a period of due diligence, he determines that he cannot treat them ethically and effectively. To do so prematurely would be discriminatory and counter to the values of the counseling profession.

IN-CLASS DISCUSSION AND EXERCISES

Group Discussion: The Art of Secret Keeping

One of the more challenging aspects of confidentiality is keeping compelling information completely secret. Specifically, the stories counselors hear on a daily basis can be both captivating and thought provoking, and not sharing specific details with friends and family can be challenging.

After reading through the cases described here, what would you describe as your most significant tripping points? What types of client stories would be difficult *not* to share with others? What specific strategies will you employ to ensure that you maintain your emotional well-being while maintaining your clients' confidence?

Group Discussion: Exceptions to the Rule

Is it okay to share client stories with your partner, spouse, or close friends who are not in the mental health field if you refrain from disclosing specific identifying information? If you or a loved one were seeking counseling services, would you feel comfortable knowing that the counselor discussed broad details sans specifics? Can you think of any exceptions where you might have no choice but to share information with friends or family (e.g., when a client approaches you in public)?

Role Play: In the Wink of an Eye

Using the scenario described in *In the Wink of an Eye*, role-play possible outcomes. Have one member play the role of Carl and two others play the roles of David and Valerie discussing the situation afterward. If you were Carl, how might you actually respond in the moment? As David, how might you actually feel or respond in the moment if Carl were to address your wink or ignore it? If you were Valerie, how would you respond to a couples counselor asking about your husband's wink in response to accusations of infidelity?

Documentation: Problem, Data, Assessment, and Plan

Using the Problem, Data, Assessment, and Plan (PDAP) format, pick one of the cases and write a progress note indicating the following:

Problem: What were the presenting concerns of this particular interaction?

Data: What, objectively, has happened? Remember to write this without subjective language or interpretation.

Assessment: As the counselor or supervisor in question, what *should* be done? Be sure to demonstrate comprehensive use of the decision-making model in this section.

Plan: What *will* be done? Be sure to outline a comprehensive plan that relates to the decision-making model.

References

Ambady, N., LaPlante, D., Nguyen, T., Rosenthal, R., Chaumeton, N., & Levinson, W. (2002). Surgeons' tone of voice: A clue to malpractice history. *Surgery, 132*(1), 5–9. doi:10.1067/msy.2002.124733

Centers for Disease Control and Prevention. (2019). *Hepatitis C questions and answers for the public.* Retrieved from https://www.cdc.gov/hepatitis/hcv/cfaq.htm#C3

Cottone, R. R. (2001). A social constructivism model of ethical decision-making in counseling. *Journal of Counseling and Development, 79*(1), 39–45. doi:10.1002/j.1556-6676.2001.tb01941.x

Forester-Miller, H., & Davis, T. E. (2016). *Practitioner's guide to ethical decision-making* (Rev. ed.). Retrieved from https://www.counseling.org/docs/default-source/ethics/practioner-39-s-guide-to-ethical-decision-making.pdf?sfvrsn=10

Jacob, C. J., Roth, G., Cliento, B., & Stoler, J. (2015). The 2014 ACA code of ethics: What's new, what's the same, and what matters for practicing clinicians. *Journal of the Pennsylvania Counseling Association, 14,* 39–46.

Kerwin, M. E., Kirby, K. C., Speziali, D., Duggan, M., Mellitz, C., Versek, B., & McNamara, A. (2015). What can parents do? A review of state laws regarding decision-making for adolescent drug abuse and mental health treatment. *Journal of Child and Adolescent Substance Abuse, 24*(3), 166–176. doi:10.1080/1067828X.2013.777380

National Institute on Drug Abuse. (2015, June 25). *Nationwide trends.* Retrieved from https://www.drugabuse.gov/publications/drugfacts/nationwide-trends

Shannon, S. K., Uggen, C., Schnittker, J., Thompson, M., Wakefield, S., & Massoglia, M. (2017). The growth, scope, and spatial distribution of people with felony records in the United States, 1948–2010. *Demography, 54*(5), 1795–1818. doi:10.1007/s13524-017-0611-1

Tarvydas, V. M. (1998). Ethical decision-making processes. In R. R. Cottone & V. M. Tarvydas (Eds.), *Ethical and professional issues in counseling* (pp. 144–155). Upper Saddle River, NJ: Prentice Hall.

Woo, J., Bhalerao, A., Bawor, M., Bhatt, M., Dennis, B., Mouravska, N., ... Samaan, Z. (2017). "Don't judge a book by its cover": A qualitative study of methadone patients' experiences of stigma. *Substance Abuse: Research and Treatment, 11,* 1–12. doi:10.1177/1178221816685087

CHAPTER 3

PROFESSIONAL RESPONSIBILITY (SECTION C OF THE ACA CODE OF ETHICS)

INTRODUCTION

Counselors are required to present both the profession and themselves to the public in a manner that engenders confidence and trust. At times, a counselor's professional responsibility can create both personal and professional challenges. This is particularly true when peers or supervisors demonstrate evidence of impairment or incompetence. The following cases outline the complications that can arise regarding counselors' efforts to monitor both their own actions and behaviors and those of their peers, colleagues, and supervisors.

All cases will be assessed using Ling and Hauck's (2017) ETHICS model for making an ethical decision.

LING AND HAUCK'S ETHICS MODEL

The ETHICS model not only takes into consideration previous decision-making models but also considers the context in which counselors are making ethical decisions. The decision-making process is founded in moral relativism, in that what constitutes acceptable morality is defined by cultural context. However, the ETHICS model considers the American Counseling Association (ACA) code as part of the first step in evaluating the dilemma, suggesting a process that is grounded in both utilitarian thought and adherence to the profession's standards. This is a more recent model and was developed after the implementation of the 2014 ACA Code of Ethics. The steps for decision-making include the following:

1. **E-Evaluate the dilemma.** Counselors first determine the nature and extent of the ethical dilemma presented by a particular case. This is the most important part of the process, as it defines the nature of the problem at the outset and requires an investigation into the code of ethics to determine its extent and potential resolutions. A dilemma typically indicates a conflict of interest of some kind, in that the needs of one involved party (the client, the counselor, or any other stakeholder) conflict with another.

2. **T-Think ahead.** Counselors then make efforts to practice mindful awareness related to any potential courses of action. At this stage, there should be—based upon the investigation into the code of ethics—some preliminary ideas about potential solutions. The goal should be to carefully consider possible

solutions, what the potential outcomes of these solutions might be, and the impact they might have on the client, the clinician, any other relevant parties, and the reputation of the profession.

3. **H-Help.** Counselors should make efforts to consult with peers and colleagues as appropriate. The governing principle is that no important decision should be made in isolation, and efforts to resolve any ethical quagmire should be no different. Per the model's progenitors, consultations in this section should be categorized as ethical, legal, clinical, or risk management.
4. **I-Information.** Counselors must obtain additional relevant information to aid in decision-making as required. This may include obtaining additional information pertaining to the dilemma itself and the involved stakeholders, though it will be important to explore relevant literature connected to the dilemma as well. Once this additional information has been obtained, the counselor needs to explore how it will affect the potential solutions devised in step 2.
5. **C-Calculate risk.** Counselors then determine the potential pros and cons of any potential courses of action selected in light of all of the information available. No decision can be made without risk, and the goal at this step is to calculate its impact on the client, the counselor, and/or any other involved stakeholders. There might also be some negotiation of risk based upon the potential solutions.
6. **S-Select an action.** Finally, counselors determine what exactly will be done and how.

BOUNDARIES OF COMPETENCE (*CAN YOU TAKE CARE OF THAT FOR US? THANKS!*)

Keri works as a lead counselor in a career counseling center at a small college and has extensive experience administering career assessments. Career assessments are a substantial part of her job, and she regularly uses them in her work with students. She is particularly well versed in using the self-directed search (SDS), which is an integral part of the career center's assessment battery.

The university has hired a new career counselor, Brittany, to work with Keri. Though Brittany has no prior experience working as a career counselor, they chose her because—per the director of the career counseling center that made the final decision to hire her—she is "intuitive and seems to be a real people person." The director decided that because of Keri's experience, she would be the perfect person to oversee Brittany during her orientation period.

Even though she interacts well with the students, it is clear to Keri that Brittany has no experience in administering the assessments that are frequently administered to students. In fact, several students have complained that Brittany has made bold claims about the utility of the SDS. One came to Keri after a session with Brittany complaining that "Brittany said the test was foolproof and that I'm supposed to be a biologist."

When Keri brought this up to her supervisor, the response was lackluster: They stated that the center has no budget for additional training, and they are requesting that Keri work with Brittany to become better acquainted with the center's assessments and procedures.

Questions for Discussion

1. *If Brittany is intending to practice under Keri's supervision as she becomes more adept at assessment instruments, is she behaving unethically?*
2. *If the administration is aware and considers this acceptable, what else can Keri do?*
3. *What kind of training would be required for Brittany to be considered competent to administer the SDS?*

Straight From the Code

1. **C.2.a. Boundaries of Competence:** Counselors practice only within the boundaries of their competence, based on their education, training, supervised experience, state and national professional credentials, and appropriate professional experience. Whereas multicultural counseling competency is required across all counseling specialties, counselors gain knowledge, personal awareness, sensitivity, dispositions, and skills pertinent to being a culturally competent counselor in working with a diverse client population.

2. **C.2.b. New Specialty Areas of Practice:** Counselors practice in specialty areas new to them only after appropriate education, training, and supervised experience. While developing skills in new specialty areas, counselors take steps to ensure the competence of their work and protect others from possible harm.

Applying a Decision-Making Model: Ling and Hauck's ETHICS Model

1. **E-Evaluate the dilemma.** A new hire, Brittany has no experience in career counseling, yet she is already seeing students and administering assessments. Not only is she ill prepared to assist the students, but she is also dispensing advice that may be directly harmful. On an organizational level, another piece of this dilemma is that the office is aware of these ethical infractions and does not seem to mind.

2. **T-Think ahead.** The primary concern in this case is the clients Brittany has been seeing. Despite (what are assumed to be) her best intentions, Brittany is giving inaccurate advice that may be confusing at best and harmful at worst. The SDS is a measure of interest and does not offer any assurances such that its findings could be considered either conclusive or foolproof (Holland & Rayman, 2013).

Though it may not be her preferred choice, Keri could concede to assisting Brittany in developing her skills; this would technically fall under the umbrella of acceptable practice on Brittany's behalf. Kerri could also refuse to work with Brittany if she feels she is incapable of providing this supervision for some reason, though this might cause friction with her employers.

3. **H-Help.** Though the primary concern is the clients being treated, Keri should also consider the needs of her colleague. While Brittany should most assuredly not be administering the SDS given her current level of understanding, she should be given the opportunity to succeed in her position by being afforded the appropriate training and support. Though Keri is identified as a lead counselor, it may be worth clarifying with her supervisors the extent to which she is responsible for training other staff members.
4. **I-Information.** Assuming Keri has any responsibility regarding Brittany's training, it would be prudent to examine how best to provide the appropriate training and ensure her competence. Specifically, what areas of missing knowledge account for Brittany's behaviors with her clients? Is it that she lacks understanding regarding the utility of the SDS? Is it that she lacks fundamental knowledge related to the function of a career counselor? Is this simply evidence of confusion regarding the difference between interest assessment and ability testing?
5. **C-Calculate risk.** The risks of *not* providing assistance to Brittany seem substantial: Brittany's behaviors are likely causing some form of harm to her clients, and refusing to supervise her could cause problems with Keri's employer. However, Keri needs to be careful about the potential liabilities inherent in overseeing Brittany's clinical work: If she is technically acting as Brittany's supervisor and Brittany were sued for malpractice for some reason, she could be liable as well (Recupero & Rainey, 2007). If she were uncomfortable with this risk, Keri should clarify with Brittany what her deficits in training are and work with her supervisor to help determine her training needs.
6. **S-Select an action.** It would be best to begin by speaking with Brittany directly to determine her needs for training and development to assist her supervisor, though Keri will have to be cautious in her approach. The goal would ultimately be to provide support and guidance by first determining her needs and then working with the center's administration to address them.

The Likely Answer

Keri should first speak with Brittany to obtain additional information regarding her struggles in implementing the SDS with students. Once she gains clarity regarding Brittany's needs, she should reach out to her supervisor to ensure that Brittany not be able to see clients (or at the very least not be permitted to administer the SDS) without additional training and supervision and to help develop a plan of action to ensure she receives this training.

RECRUITING THROUGH EMPLOYMENT (*YOU CAN'T TAKE THEM WITH YOU*)

Fred has been working in a community mental health agency for several years and really enjoys his work. However, he has decided he wants to own his own practice and is preparing to transition out of the agency to private practice full time.

Just so no one is caught completely off guard, he has been letting his clients know that he will be leaving at the end of the month. Although excited, Fred is also nervous about the change since he knows gaining clients can be much more difficult when he is on his own in private practice.

In the interest of embracing the entrepreneurial spirit of his new endeavor, Fred has devised a plan: For his current clients, instead of letting them know their case will be transferred, he plans to suggest that it would be best if they stayed with him in his new practice. He is also planning to offer to give them two free sessions for transferring over to his practice as an extra incentive. He hopes that the financial deal coupled with not wanting to restart a relationship with a new counselor should help give him some clients and ease some of his worries.

Questions for Discussion

1. *Though Fred's plan is a savvy business strategy, is it ethically sound?*
2. *If clients ask to follow Fred to his practice without his prompting, is it acceptable for him to take them?*
3. *Are there better ways for Fred to generate business for his practice?*

Straight From the Code

1. **C.3.d. Recruiting Through Employment:** Counselors do not use their places of employment or institutional affiliation to recruit clients, supervisors, or consultees for their private practices.

Applying a Decision-Making Model: Ling and Hauck's ETHICS Model

1. **E-Evaluate the dilemma.** Fred is using his place of employment to springboard his caseload for his private practice. Not only is he trying

to funnel business to his new endeavor, but he also is offering financial incentives for his clients to make the switch.

2. **T-Think ahead.** Fred's offer to have his clients transition to his new practice is not in and of itself a violation of ethics. In fact, it would be appropriate to inform his clients well in advance of his change in employment and provide them with options moving forward (with the decision to follow him among them). The major concern in this case is that if Fred makes an offer for discounted rates as a function of treatment decisions, he is engaging in coercion.

3. **H-Help.** Fred's primary concern should be his client's well-being, though this situation highlights the conflict that can occur between defining a client's needs in contrast to a counselor's needs. Fred needs to keep a steady flow of income, but he also needs to ensure that his clients have autonomy regarding their course of treatment. Consultation is critical in all ethical dilemmas, though this situation, in particular, may warrant careful examination of the consultant; specifically, Fred needs to be careful not to simply consult with peers or supervisors that will support his financial concerns.

4. **I-Information.** Fred needs to consider if there are any stipulations in his contract at his agency that forbid him from "poaching" clients for his private practice. It is not uncommon for agencies and group practices to include a noncompete clause as a part of a hiring package. In these cases, the employee has signed a legally binding document indicating that he or she will not enter into or start a practice that directly competes with his or her employer's business.

5. **C-Calculate risk.** If Fred offers this financial enticement to his clients, he is incentivizing the continuation of a service that may or may not be in their best interest. He may also be violating his contract of employment and is certainly violating the code of ethics. However, he needs to inform his clients of his decision to leave and afford them the option to choose their own course of action regarding their continued treatment.

6. **S-Select an Action.** Fred should certainly inform his clients of his decision to leave and may even inform them of his new practice location. However, he has to be certain that their decision to continue with treatment is their own.

The Likely Answer

Fred should give his clients advance notice of his new location and explain that they are free to follow him there or to accept referrals to other providers in the area that he will happily provide.

EXPLOITATION OF OTHERS (*EVERYONE GETS THEIR 15 MINUTES*)

Liam, a counselor in a community mental health center with a high volume, is struggling financially. Incentives and bonuses for staff at this agency are based on revenue: The more money you bring in to the center, the more you get paid. To help his chances at a bonus for this quarter, he is seeing clients for 45 minutes but is in fact billing his clients' insurance companies for 60 minutes as this permits him to earn about $15 more per session. He also tries to use the extra time to catch up on his progress notes.

Recently, one of Liam's clients asked Liam's supervisor (Tayz) if 45 minutes is the standard session length, as she heard other patients see their counselors for 60 minutes. Tayz then calls Liam in to ask about the discrepancies in client reports and his documentation.

Questions for Discussion

1. *As Liam's supervisor, how should Tayz respond?*
2. *What are the consequences for the client not receiving 60 minutes?*
3. *Are there any legal ramifications for falsifying how much time is spent with a client directly?*

Straight From the Code

1. **C.6.d. Exploitation of Others:** Counselors do not exploit others in their professional relationships.
2. **C.2.e. Consultations on Ethical Obligations:** Counselors take reasonable steps to consult with other counselors, the ACA Ethics and Professional Standards Department, or related professionals when they have questions regarding their ethical obligations or professional practice.

Applying a Decision-Making Model: Ling and Hauck's ETHICS Model

1. **E-Evaluate the dilemma.** Liam's financial concerns may be serious, but they are only going to get worse if he finds himself or his employer under investigation for insurance fraud. A counselor billing for a 60-minute session when he or she has only provided 45 minutes is both unethical and illegal. Now that Tayz is aware of this, he needs to notify the insurance companies implicated, but he may worry about the impact this will have on the center.

2. **T-Think ahead.** One concern Tayz may have in notifying the insurance companies is further deception: Liam could lie and state that he has been seeing clients for 60 minutes, as it would be the client's word versus his. Liam might edit also all of his nonbilled documentation to reflect the correct hours. He could also review all his documentation and ensure correct time stamps. Tayz may also be concerned about the impact this will have on the center and/or his career; specifically, if the center is sanctioned for this discrepancy, Tayz may be shooting himself in the foot professionally and financially.

3. **H-Help.** Regardless of these concerns, Tayz is obligated to ensure the welfare of clients treated by any clinician under his supervision. Liam's actions are not just a violation of the code; he is technically stealing money relegated to health insurance costs contributed by his clients and their insurers. It will be important for him to consult first with a supervisor at the center, but he may also wish to reach out to a colleague *not* affiliated with the center in the hopes of obtaining an unbiased perspective.

4. **I-Information.** Tayz should check with either his direct supervisor or the center's human resources division to determine what protocols are to be followed. He may need to consult with local law enforcement as well, as Liam's actions are likely in violation of state (if not national) law.

5. **C-Calculate risk.** The risks in notifying the insurance companies affected by Liam's actions are—as stated earlier—mostly related to the possibility of continued deception on behalf of Liam. Though the risk to the center's continued existence may be a concern, it cannot be a deciding factor when a clinician is engaged in a crime that defrauds clients as well as the public. Additionally, the risk inherent in *not* reporting is likely greater with regard to the impact it could have on the center's clients.

6. **S-Select an action.** Tayz likely has no choice but to escalate these concerns through the appropriate channels at the center. Depending on protocol as established by his employers and the related insurance companies, he may have to file a police report as well.

The Likely Answer

Tayz should first verify that there is evidence to indicate that Liam falsified his documentation, consult with his supervisor and/or human resources division regarding protocol, and notify the insurance companies implicated and/or law enforcement regarding what has occurred.

EFFECTIVENESS AND IMPAIRMENT (UN-*HAPPY HOUR*)

Mary and Tony work together as counselors in a partial hospital program for children. Mary has been employed there for 1 year, and Tony for a little longer. Since they were hired around the same time, they have a fairly close relationship. They even go to happy hour once a week together, though Mary has noticed that Tony is drinking a little more than usual during these outings as of late.

During their last get-together, Tony had a few too many cocktails and had to catch a rideshare home. Just before he left, he shared with Mary that he is divorcing his wife. He was tearful in describing the separation and seemed pretty broken up about it. When she watched him get in his ride, the last thing he said to her was "I just can't stand not seeing my kids," with tears streaming down his face.

Unfortunately, the problem goes beyond the excessive drinking during happy hour: During the past month, Mary notices Tony has started to look disheveled when arriving at work, at times seems to smell of alcohol (though she is not certain of this), and has been coming in 20 to 30 minutes late every day. Mary is worried about his mental health but is also concerned for the safety of the children in the program.

Questions for Discussion

1. *Should Mary discuss the issue directly with Tony, or should she reach out directly to her supervisor?*
2. *What are the potential legal issues involved in Tony's actions?*
3. *Does Mary have the right to discuss these concerns with her coworkers?*

Straight From the Code

1. **C.2.d. Monitor Effectiveness:** Counselors continually monitor their effectiveness as professionals and take steps to improve when necessary. Counselors take reasonable steps to seek peer supervision to evaluate their efficacy as counselors.

2. **C.2.g. Impairment:** Counselors monitor themselves for signs of impairment from their own physical, mental, or emotional problems and refrain from offering or providing professional services when impaired. They seek assistance for problems that reach the level of professional impairment, and, if necessary, they limit, suspend, or terminate their professional responsibilities until it is determined that they may safely resume their work. Counselors assist colleagues or supervisors in recognizing their own professional impairment and provide consultation and assistance when warranted with colleagues or supervisors showing signs of impairment and intervene as appropriate to prevent imminent harm to clients.

Applying a Decision-Making Model: Ling and Hauck's ETHICS Model

1. **E-Evaluate the dilemma.** Mary is concerned about Tony's effectiveness as a counselor in addition to his well-being. In order to keep clients at the program safe, Mary *could* report Tony's current state to her supervisor; however, as Tony's friend and colleague, Mary is likely also worried about the potential ramifications this report could have on his career, his mental health, and their friendship. Additionally, aside from his being late, the case does not indicate that Mary has witnessed Tony harming clients in any way (directly or indirectly), as her concerns about drinking on the job are speculative.

2. **T-Think ahead.** Again, Mary could certainly justify going over Tony's head and expressing concern to his supervisor. However, this would likely have detrimental outcomes for Tony (particularly if he is reprimanded in some way), not to mention their friendship. She could reach out to Tony directly and express her concerns, though this is likely to be a difficult conversation that could also affect their friendship.

3. **H-Help.** Reaching out to a colleague is probably the best place to start in seeking guidance or support, though Mary will have to carefully consider whether she wants to speak with someone who knows Tony and/or is involved with the hospital or someone else whose perspective is less biased. For the latter, it would make sense to solicit an unbiased perspective, but it might also be beneficial to speak with a colleague who knows Tony and the specifics of his situation.

4. **I-Information.** Again, Mary has no information to indicate that Tony is putting his clients in direct harm, but she does have information indicating that he is struggling in some way. A reasonable place to begin would be to determine if there is evidence to suggest Tony's clients have been placed in some form of risk, though this would be difficult to obtain without speaking to a supervisor (or Tony's clients, which is likely an inappropriate course of action). She might also just directly ask Tony if he has been drinking on the job, though she would have no guarantees regarding the honesty of his answer.

   It might also be helpful to explore what (if any) policies and procedures exist within the hospital regarding employee health and safety. The goal would be to find resources that she could offer to Tony in addition to determining what sort of procedures are in place regarding the management of impaired clinicians. There may be an employee assistance program that Mary could refer Tony to, or perhaps some other form of counseling or support is offered to employees.

5. **C-Calculate risk.** Mary's primary dilemma is whether to simply talk to Tony and express her concerns or to discuss the matter with his

supervisor. Unfortunately for Mary, this is an all too common problem, as research suggests that most counselors in practice are aware of or work directly with impaired colleagues (Brown-Rice & Furr, 2015). However, Mary needs to be careful in her response: If she reports Tony, this might actually make things worse as it could harm their friendship and could affect his job, but she could be sure that all involved are aware of the problem. If she decides to only discuss the matter with Tony, she may have a better chance of effecting change, but she is withholding information from her employer regarding an impaired colleague.

6. **S-Select an action.** It would be helpful for Mary to first discuss the matter with two colleagues—perhaps one who knows Tony and/or works for the hospital and another who does not. Depending on the feedback she receives, it might be best to begin by discussing her concerns with Tony directly and waiting to refer that matter to a higher level until she has more information indicating that Tony's clients are being affected in some way.

The Likely Answer

Mary should check in with Tony, provide her support as a friend, and recommend that he seek help from a professional counselor (either independently or through the hospital's human resources department). If he is unwilling to do so, she should discuss the matter with his supervisor. If he is willing to do so, she should leave the matter for now and discuss the matter with his supervisor if his condition persists or further deteriorates.

NONDISCRIMINATION (*HOW DO I MAKE THIS RIGHT?*)

Barry has been working as the only high school counselor for several years in a small rural school district with predominately Latino/a/x students. Most—if not all—of the students are first-generation college students, whereas some are also considered undocumented students and have limited English proficiency.

He receives notification of a large financial scholarship for first-generation Latino/a/x students who plan on going to a local state university. The only requirements of the scholarship are "students must be first generation and Latino." The scholarship's application does not ask other questions such as immigration status or language proficiency. Barry knows he is not permitted to ask his students of their immigrant status, but he does have access to copies of birth certificates and language proficiency. He has often had to review these documents for other duties. He also has access to grade point averages, coursework, and test scores.

Barry decides that instead of gathering more information, he is only going to select a few students who will be informed about applying for this scholarship. He chooses five male students who he knows well and believes to be good candidates. However, he also selects these individuals as he remembers they have U.S. birth certificates and are not receiving English as a second language service. He contacts them individually and agrees to assist them with the application process.

A week after notifying these students, Barry is torn. He initially saw no issue with this decision, but he now worries that his actions were in fact an act of discrimination. Specifically, he is no longer certain that he chose students based on merit and is worried that he instead was influenced by his bias in favor of individuals born in the United States as opposed to those born in Mexico or Guatemala.

Questions for Discussion

1. *As Barry let only U.S.-born male Latino students know about scholarship, is this considered discrimination?*
2. *Knowing how labor intensive it is, should Barry have gone through all files and let all the students and genders who are listed as Latino/a/x know about the scholarship?*
3. *What should Barry do now that select students have been notified?*

Straight From the Code

1. **C.5. Nondiscrimination:** Counselors do not condone or engage in discrimination against prospective or current clients, students, employees, supervisees, or research participants based on age, culture, disability, ethnicity, race, religion/spirituality, gender, gender identity, sexual orientation, marital/partnership status, language preference, socioeconomic status, immigration status, or any basis proscribed by law.

Applying a Decision-Making Model: Ling and Hauck's ETHICS Model

1. **E-Evaluate the dilemma.** Barry was aware of a scholarship available to all first-generation Latino students, regardless of gender, immigration status, and/or language proficiency. Barry knew it would take a great deal of time to look through all student files to gather additional information, so he opted to use a combination of intuition and personal values to make a difficult decision. He is now torn between accepting this decision for what it was or making some effort to remedy what may have been an act of bias and/or discrimination.
2. **T-Think ahead.** Barry selecting students based on his beliefs about their individual abilities is not necessarily a violation of any ethical code, since providing students with scholarship information is a

form of advocacy and often part of the role of the school counselor. The concern is who are being excluded (and how) in his selection. Barry might see his decision to select certain students as an example of beneficence by helping those *he* believes are deserving students to have access to a scholarship. However, this negates the ethical principle of justice, since the decision not to consider all students is neither fair nor equitable.

This type of bias in decision-making is not uncommon (Koch, D'Mello, & Sackett, 2015), and concerns regarding the equitable treatment of Latinx students in academic settings are significant throughout the United States (McWhirter, Garcia, & Bines, 2018). Though it is highly unlikely that he acted with malicious intent, Barry is still obligated to respond in some way. That he made a mistake or error in judgment is not the presenting problem; how he responds moving forward is the primary concern, and the fair treatment of all students is essential.

3. **H-Help.** In this case, solid decision-making is unlikely to occur in isolation, and Barry should definitely consult with a peer to help make a decision about what the next course of action should be. Whom to ask for advice or guidance is less clear, as he would need to be assured that any individual provides the necessary feedback rather than the feedback that would make Barry feel less guilty (or exacerbate his anxieties unnecessarily) about his actions. Barry could seek assistance from a colleague, though this presents the risk inherent in having a friend provide supportive (rather than critical) feedback. Though representatives at the school may respond punitively if they believe Barry acted unethically, he could reach out to a school administrator to see about policies and what should be done. He could also contact the sponsor of the scholarship to gather further details on the requirements, to make sure he is practicing within the regulations of the award.

4. **I-Information.** Barry needs to consider the information provided in the scholarship and what types of information he had access to during his initial decisions. Upon retrospect, is he able to clearly delineate how and why he made the selections that he did?

5. **C-Calculate risk.** Barry may run the risk of being penalized by his school and its administration if he explains to them his concerns that he erred in providing scholarship support to some students and not others. However, if Barry continues to exclude students based on gender, immigration status, and language proficiency, the fact that deserving students are being denied a scholarship is a significant risk to the well-being of the clients he serves. He is violating the Code of Ethics and is at risk for losing his job, school counseling certification, not to mention a potential discrimination lawsuit.

6. **S-Select an action.** Barry seems to have little recourse beyond discussing the matter directly with the administration at the school or his direct supervisor and may face consequences for his initial decisions. However, there may still be a chance that eligible students could apply (it has only been a week since notifications were sent out), and the potential risk to clients and the profession of *not* doing so is substantial.

The Likely Answer

Barry should reach out to the scholarship to determine exactly what the parameters of the scholarship are and what deadlines currently exist. He should then report to his supervisor his concerns about potential bias in his decision-making and determine collaboratively what next steps should entail.

CREDENTIALS, DEGREES, AND IMPLICATIONS OF COMPETENCE (*YOU SAY POTATO, I SAY COUNSELOR*)

Quyntyn is a counselor in private practice. As he values his own well-being—both in general and as it pertains to the support he provides his clients—he has decided to enter into individual counseling to address stress in his work and personal life. He has been established with an individual counselor that he has seen on and off for years now, but—much to his chagrin—he finds that she has retired and is unwilling to schedule additional appointments.

After a quick search on the Internet, he finds Jean-Baptiste, a counselor and psychologist in the area who specializes in existential psychotherapy (this is right up Quyntyn's alley). He schedules an appointment with Jean-Baptiste: They meet, he feels like they click, and he agrees to set up another appointment.

In the time between these appointments, however, Quyntyn notices some points of concern in Jean-Baptiste's consent form that he took home with him. When Quyntyn did an Internet search to verify his credentials, he is surprised to find that Jean-Baptiste is in fact *not* a licensed psychologist as indicated in his promotional material. He does hold a doctoral degree in counselor education and is a licensed professional counselor, but he refers to himself as a "licensed counseling psychologist" despite not having a degree in psychology or licensure as a psychologist.

Questions for Discussion

1. *As the distinction in terminology is very subtle (i.e., counselor versus counseling psychologist), has Jean-Baptiste committed an ethical violation in this case?*

2. *As Quyntyn is a client and not a colleague, is he obligated to respond in any way?*
3. *If Quyntyn did choose to respond in some fashion, should he first discuss the matter with Jean-Baptiste directly?*

Straight From the Code

1. **C.4.a. Accurate Representation.** Counselors claim or imply only professional qualifications actually completed and correct any known misrepresentations of their qualifications by others. Counselors truthfully represent the qualifications of their professional colleagues. Counselors clearly distinguish between paid and volunteer work experience and accurately describe their continuing education and specialized training.

2. **C.4.b. Credentials.** Counselors claim only licenses or certifications that are current and in good standing.

3. **C.4.c. Educational Degrees.** Counselors clearly differentiate between earned and honorary degrees.

Applying a Decision-Making Model: Ling and Hauck's ETHICS Model

1. **E-Evaluate the dilemma.** Ethical dilemmas can occur anytime and anywhere, though it is unfortunate that Quyntyn should have to consider something of this nature when he is simply trying to get support. However, he now knows that his counselor—whom he feels a connection with and would likely have continued to see without concern for his competence had he not conducted an Internet search—is indeed misrepresenting his credentials to the public. He now has to decide if this concern warrants an action of some kind.

2. **T-Think ahead.** The first option for Quyntyn is to say nothing at all and simply continue seeing Jean-Baptiste for counseling. This would certainly be appropriate in his role as a client, but it would negate his concerns as a professional counselor that provides services to the very same public that Jean-Baptiste is defrauding. He could address the matter directly with Jean-Baptiste, but this would run the risk of damaging a relationship with a counselor that he feels a connection with during a time of personal need. Another option would be to file an anonymous report with the state licensing board; this would address his concerns but could be very damaging to Jean-Baptiste.

3. **H-Help.** Thankfully, Quyntyn is free to consult with whomever he pleases in this case: Any colleague in the mental health profession

would suffice, though he might also want to consult with associates *outside* the mental health profession. Specifically, what would individuals not affiliated with the world of mental health think and feel if they were in Quyntyn's shoes?

4. **I-Information.** Quyntyn might want to further investigate Jean-Baptiste's promotional materials, particularly via the Internet. Is this simply a typo on a standard office form, or is this a consistent pattern of misrepresentation? Quyntyn might also want to reach out to the state licensing board to determine what the potential consequences of misrepresenting credentials are in his state.

5. **C-Calculate risk.** If Quyntyn chooses to say and do nothing, this could likely be to his benefit as a client (assuming he can ignore his concerns about Jean-Baptiste's actions). However, the risk to the integrity of the respective professions of counseling and psychology might be difficult to ignore, as this denigrates both: Psychologists have a different set of licensing standards, and counselors have a storied history of efforts to maintain reputability as an independent profession (see Ponton & Duba, 2009). If Quyntyn finds that this is a consistent pattern of misrepresentation, he might feel most comfortable confronting Jean-Baptiste directly, though this will likely have an impact on their counseling relationship.

6. **S-Select an action.** Quyntyn is not acting as a counselor in this capacity, and he is certainly within his right to say and do nothing if he chooses. However, addressing his concern with Jean-Baptiste is likely the most ethical course of action.

The Likely Answer

Quyntyn should begin by searching through Jean-Baptiste's promotional materials to determine if this is a consistent pattern or a one-time misnomer. In either case, he should next mention his concerns to Jean-Baptiste. He should likely escalate the matter to the state's licensing board if this misrepresentation is consistent throughout his promotional materials and Jean-Baptiste declines to address the matter.

PERSONAL PUBLIC STATEMENTS (*IS THIS THING ON?*)

Aleister is a counselor educator in a tenure-track position at a state university. He is getting his materials ready for tenure and promotion and is looking to boost his reputation as an expert in the field. Lucky for him, he knows one of the administrators for a local radio station who hosts a weekly call-in show and secures a spot on a segment related to mental health titled *Who's who and what matters in the world of mental health.* He has been asked to provide an overview of the differences between counselors, psychologists, social workers, and psychiatrists, as well as field questions from callers looking for advice in seeking mental health treatment.

On the day of the broadcast, Aleister is in top form! He provides a concise overview of the professions and successfully fields a couple of questions from callers about their efforts to find supportive counseling for themselves and their family members. He even manages a few bits of playful banter with the host.

Right before his segment ends, however, the host sets him up to comment about the president's current policies toward mental health. Aleister—still running hot from his success with the show and having fun with the interview—makes a joke about the president as being "reviled" by mental health professionals and counselors, in particular.

His comment gets a laugh from the host and the others in the studio, and the segment ends. Immediately, Aleister worries that he overstepped a boundary, but he is unsure what (if anything) can be done.

Questions for Discussion

1. *Is it ever appropriate for a counselor to make public statements about their political beliefs or affiliations?*
2. *Would it have been more acceptable for Aleister to indicate his political beliefs were not representative of the profession as a whole?*
3. *What should Aleister do now? The program has ended; should he ask for a correction of some kind?*

Straight From the Code

1. **C.8.a. Personal Public Statements.** When making personal statements in a public context, counselors clarify that they are speaking from their personal perspectives and that they are not speaking on behalf of all counselors or the profession.

Applying a Decision-Making Model: Ling and Hauck's ETHICS Model

1. **E-Evaluate the dilemma.** Aleister is certainly entitled to his own political beliefs, and there is little in the Code to suggest that he is unable to support specific political candidates. However, his comment at the end of the program did not indicate a personal affiliation; he claimed—in the context of a joke—that he spoke for the entire profession in his opinions of a specific politician. While the program is over, he is still faced with the concern that he overstepped his professional boundaries and made broad claims about the profession in general.

2. **T-Think ahead.** The first option for Aleister is to say nothing at all and simply hope that no one expresses concerns about his statement. While this may be tempting, it denies him the chance to make this situation right, as he was objectively wrong in his statement (i.e., he cannot say conclusively that the entire profession is in alignment with his political views). Another option would be to ask the station to issue a correction or a retraction, but this will likely cause some amount of harm to his reputation.
3. **H-Help.** In the moment, Aleister has few options with regard to consultation. However, he is certainly able to consult with peers and colleagues after the show has concluded. If anything, it might be useful to consult with a variety of professional counselors—those who know him well and those whom he trusts—to see if they have any sense of what should be considered moving forward.
4. **I-Information.** In the moment, Aleister should ask the station if there is any option to issue a retraction. He should—at the very least—have a clear indication as to what options exist regarding the correction of statements made during a public broadcast.
5. **C-Calculate risk.** If Aleister simply waits to see if there is any fallout from his statements, he runs the risk of missing an opportunity to correct a public statement that he knew immediately to be false. If he chooses to pursue a public correction of some kind, he may damage his reputation both publicly and with the station with which he now has a working relationship.
6. **S-Select an action.** Though it will likely be difficult to do so, Aleister should make an effort to issue a retraction of some kind.

The Likely Answer

As soon as Aleister is aware of his misstep, he should ask the station what options exist regarding a retraction of his statement. To be certain this is required, he should also consult with peers and colleagues regarding the content of his statement to be certain this warrants a retraction.

IN-CLASS DISCUSSION AND EXERCISES

Group Discussion: Keeping Our Biases in Check

Cases such as *Everyone Gets Their 15 Minutes* highlight the degree of difficulty inherent in negotiating financial needs with clinical needs. Specifically, clinicians and supervisors are often faced with difficult choices related to treatment needs that have an impact on their financial bottom line. In private practice, it can be challenging for any clinician to determine with certainty that their decisions related to client treatment are motivated by clinical acumen or their mortgage payment.

Imagine that you are in a position where a colleague—whose sole source of income is their private practice—has asked you to help determine if he or she should keep seeing a client or advocate for termination. What questions would you want your colleague to consider? How would you help guide his or her own thinking to an equitable decision? How would you advise a colleague in his or her efforts to hold personal biases lightly?

Group Discussion: Exceptions to the Rule

Cases such as Un-*happy Hour* highlight some of the ambiguity inherent in determining when a clinician is demonstrating behavior that is harmful versus potentially harmful, and the complications inherent in determining when to support versus when to report. Not discussing concerns with supervisors runs the risk of missing an opportunity to keep a client out of harm's way, but reporting every concern creates a work environment for counselors that is devoid of humanism and unlikely to promote honesty.

Where does the line exist between counselors behaving unethically and counselors struggling the way that all human beings do from time to time? If a counselor has recently suffered a loss, for example, and has asked that he or she be permitted to return to work despite demonstrating evidence of depression, does this not run the risk of potential harm to clients? By contrast, would it be appropriate to deny a counselor the opportunity to continue working as a means of maintaining his or her own mental health?

Role Play: Can You Take Care of That for Us? Thanks!

Using the scenario described in *Can You Take Care of That for Us? Thanks!*, role-play possible outcomes. Have one member play the role of Brittany and another play the role of Keri discussing the situation. If you were Keri, how might you actually respond in the moment? As Brittany, how might you actually feel or respond in the moment if you were presented with concerns about your competence? If you were Keri, how would you respond to what you likely perceive as incompetence?

Documentation: Problem, Data, Assessment, and Plan

Using the Problem, Data, Assessment, and Plan (PDAP) format, pick one of the cases and write a progress note indicating the following:

Problem: What were the presenting concerns of this particular interaction?

Data: What, objectively, has happened? Remember to write this without subjective language or interpretation.

Assessment: As the counselor or supervisor in question, what *should* be done? Be sure to demonstrate comprehensive use of the decision-making model in this section.

Plan: What *will* be done? Be sure to outline a comprehensive plan that relates to the decision-making model.

References

Brown-Rice, K., & Furr, S. (2015). Gatekeeping ourselves: Counselor educators' knowledge of colleagues' problematic behaviors. *Counselor Education and Supervision, 54*(3), 176–188. doi:10.1002/ceas.12012

Holland, J. L., & Rayman, J. R. (2013). Self-directed search. In W. B. Walsh & S. H. Osipow (Eds.), *Advances in vocational psychology: The assessment of interests* (pp. 55–82). Hillsdale, NJ: Erlbaum.

Koch, A. J., D'Mello, S. D., & Sackett, P. R. (2015). A meta-analysis of gender stereotypes and bias in experimental simulations of employment decision making. *Journal of Applied Psychology, 100*(1), 128–161. doi:10.1037/a0036734

McWhirter, E. H., Garcia, E. A., & Bines, D. (2018). Discrimination and other education barriers, school connectedness, and thoughts of dropping out among Latina/o students. *Journal of Career Development, 45*(4), 330–344. doi:10.1177/0894845317696807

Ponton, R. F., & Duba, J. D. (2009). The ACA code of ethics: Articulating counseling's professional covenant. *Journal of Counseling and Development, 87*(1), 117–121. doi:10.1002/j.1556-6678.2009.tb00557.x

Recupero, P. R., & Rainey, S. E. (2007). Liability and risk management in outpatient psychotherapy supervision. *Journal of the American Academy of Psychiatry and the Law, 35*(2), 188–195.

CHAPTER 4

RELATIONSHIPS WITH OTHER PROFESSIONALS (SECTION D OF THE ACA CODE OF ETHICS)

INTRODUCTION

Counselors' relationships with other professionals are almost as important as their relationships with their clients. Though these associations can at times be complex, managing them is critical to the profession's continued existence. The scenarios in this section focus on the personal and professional interactions between counselors and other mental health professionals.

All cases will be assessed using Corey, Corey, Corey, and Callanan's (2015) eight-step sequence for making an ethical decision.

COREY, COREY, COREY, AND CALLANAN'S MODEL

Corey, Corey, Corey, and Callanan (2015) have developed and revised a practice-based, ethical, decision-making model by integrating theory and practice-based approaches into a linear eight-step approach. Building upon notions advanced by the feminist and transcultural ethical decision-making models (as well as social constructivist concepts), they outline eight steps for counselors to consider in resolving an ethical dilemma in a manner meeting the client's best interest:

1. **Identify the problem or dilemma.** Identify the nature and scope of the presented dilemma. Counselors need to gather information during this step and should consult with all involved stakeholders to obtain as much insight as possible.

2. **Identify the potential issues involved.** Specifically, what potential conflicts exist among the needs of the client, the needs of the profession, and the needs of the clinician(s) in this case? Broader cultural needs and concerns should be considered during this step as well.

3. **Review the relevant ethics codes.** Counselors are expected to reference the code of ethics directly in the moment that decision-making takes place or in the aftermath of a decision to determine its adherence to ethical standards.

4. **Know the applicable laws and regulations.** In addition to the code of ethics, counselors should be aware of relevant state and national laws related to dilemmas as applicable. At times, conflicts may exist between state or national law and the values of the profession.

5. **Obtain consultation.** Consultation can be with supervisors or other peers in the mental health field. The goal should ultimately be to consult with colleagues who are unbiased with regard to the dilemma at hand.

6. **Consider possible and probable courses of action.** Counselors should develop a list of possible methods for resolving the dilemma.

7. **Enumerate and consider the possible consequences of various decisions.** With regard to the list developed in step 6, pros and cons for each possible option should be considered.

8. **Choose what appears to be the best course of action.** Determine what exactly will be done and how.

This model entails both the intrapsychic consideration on the part of the practitioner and the relational component of consultation. As the model has evolved, it suggests—similar to the feminist approach—that counselors should include the client whenever possible and that—similar to the transcultural integrative model—cultural differences and contexts should be considered as well.

DIFFERENT APPROACHES (*HANDS OFF MY CLIENTS!*)

Alena is a counselor struggling to develop her own private practice. She worked in a community mental health setting part time for 4 years while she completed her required hours for licensure, all the while dreaming of a future where she could be her own boss and set her own schedule. Alena loves the work with her clients, but referrals have been difficult to come by, as there are a lot of therapists in the area where she is practicing.

One of Alena's clients—Ahmir—has been seeing her for the past 2 months to address issues of depression and anxiety connected to his marriage. At Alena's suggestion, Ahmir has decided to begin couples counseling sessions with a social worker—another private practitioner in the area named Iola—that a colleague recommended.

After an initial appointment with Iola, Ahmir calls Alena to tell her that he will not be returning. He says that he met with Iola for a consultation to discuss couples counseling and that they mutually decided he would forego couples work so he could instead see her individually. He casually tells Alena that he has signed a release and that he would love for Alena to speak with Iola to "give her the rundown on what we've talked about so far."

When Alena calls Iola, she is surprised by Iola's cavalier attitude. Iola apologizes for "poaching a client" but says that it happens often. Specifically, Iola states that she makes a point to meet with members of a couple individually but that "they find my approach and my style so captivating that a lot of them just decide to stay on as individual clients."

Questions for Discussion

1. *Did Iola do anything wrong in this case?*
2. *Should Alena attempt to follow up with Ahmir in any way?*
3. *Assuming Alena is frustrated with Iola's practice in this case, is it appropriate for her to say anything?*

Straight From the Code

1. **D.1.a. Different Approaches.** Counselors are respectful of approaches that are grounded in theory and/or have an empirical or scientific foundation but may differ from their own. Counselors acknowledge the expertise of other professional groups and are respectful of their practices.

Applying a Decision-Making Model: Corey, Corey, Corey, and Callanan's Model

1. **Identify the problem or dilemma.** Iola met with a client for couples counseling who was already seeing a counselor for individual counseling. Ahmir is well within his right to see whichever clinician he chooses, but Alena might have concerns about the ethics of Iola's business and clinical practice in this case, particularly as she is now short another source of revenue.

2. **Identify the potential issues involved.** Iola identifies as a social worker, which means that her practice must meet the ethical standards of the National Association of Social Workers (NASW, 2017). As per the American Counseling Association (ACA) Code of Ethics, the NASW also states that social workers must practice within their scope of competence. As such, it may be that Iola did nothing wrong, particularly if she can demonstrate competence as both an individual and a family therapist. As standards for most social worker training programs that would result in independent licensure include coursework devoted to individual counseling (Council on Social Work Education, 2015), competence to treat an individual is unlikely to be an issue.

3. **Review the relevant ethics codes.** Unfortunately for Alena, the code of ethics for counselors and the code of ethics for social workers both do not say anything about "client poaching." Iola's decision to see clients individually for assessment purposes is an accepted practice in many approaches to couples counseling, and it is often recommended

with couples work, as individual assessments can be a useful screening tool for domestic violence (Jacob, 2013). Unless Alena has solid evidence suggesting that Iola made false claims about the efficacy of treatment or is otherwise providing a treatment that is demonstrated to cause harm to her client, it seems unlikely that a specific tenet of any code of ethics has been violated here.

However, the language in the ACA Code of Ethics does encourage that Alena be "respectful" of an approach to treatment that differs from her own. It could be inferred that being respectful of other approaches would include approaches to treatment that do not benefit Alena financially.

4. **Know the applicable laws and regulations.** Again, there is nothing in regulations for social workers, counselors, or family therapists suggesting Iola has violated any laws or regulations here.

5. **Obtain consultation.** This would be an important step, as Alena could likely use validation for her feelings of frustration. While Iola ostensibly did not violate any ethical code, her behavior could have been more collegial, and Alena has every right to be upset.

6. **Consider possible and probable courses of action.** Alena could express her frustrations with Iola, or she could simply accept the loss and move on.

7. **Enumerate and consider the possible consequences of various decisions.** It would probably feel validating for Alena to vent her frustrations to Iola, but it is unlikely that it would have any impact on the present situation. Ahmir deserves autonomy, and it was his choice to end treatment with Alena. Additionally, it is difficult to imagine an outcome of this discussion that would appease Alena's needs entirely but would also *not* violate the autonomy of her clients in some way. For example, Alena could not tell Iola that Iola is not allowed to see her clients for couples counseling. Alena also cannot tell Iola that she is not permitted to see couples for individual work or to inhibit her clients' ability in any way to see the counselor that they prefer.

8. **Choose what appears to be the best course of action.** Unfortunately for Alena, it seems as if the best course of action is to simply support Ahmir's decision to see Iola and help to facilitate the transition in a way that is civil and respectful despite her frustrations.

The Likely Answer

Alena should wish Ahmir the best, be helpful in providing Iola with any relevant treatment data requested by way of Ahmir's release, and then vent about this with her supervisor.

WORKPLACE POLICIES (*COUNSELORS UNITE!*)

Mitzi is the clinical supervisor at a community mental health center. She is new in her role, and she ascended the corporate hierarchy very quickly. Five years ago, she was completing her internship at this site while finishing her master's degree. She was hired as a counselor right after she graduated, and she was promoted to a supervisory role 2 years later once she completed her required hours for licensure.

Mitzi oversees a staff of 10 clinicians, who have all been at the site longer than she has. In fact, one of the staff members whom she oversees—Thelma—was her clinical supervisor during her internship. To put it mildly, Thelma was *livid* when Mitzi was promoted as supervisor, but Thelma's track record of difficulty with the administration has been her professional undoing. However, Thelma has a good rapport with the other counselors on staff.

As a new financial quarter approaches, Mitzi is disheartened to have to report to the staff that there will be a freeze on retirement plan matching due to overarching financial problems at the center. Though Mitzi is in no way directly responsible for this decision, she is required to tell all of her supervisees, all of whom are furious. She discusses this during a weekly group supervision meeting, and—despite anticipating a vitriolic response—she is surprised by how angry everyone is. She is particularly stunned by Thelma's role in fueling this acrimony.

Shortly after this meeting, she receives an email from Thelma (with all of her supervisees cc'd) indicating that the counselors on staff have decided to unionize. They are referring to themselves as T.U.T. (Therapist Unity Team) and are threatening to strike if retirement plans are frozen.

Questions for Discussion

1. *Are counselors permitted to unionize? Should Mitzi do anything to prevent this from happening?*
2. *Assuming the company cannot meet T.U.T.'s demands, what should Mitzi do to make sure the clinic stays operational?*
3. *Is there anything Mitzi could have done to prevent this from happening?*

Straight From the Code

1. **D.1.g. Employer Policies.** The acceptance of employment in an agency or institution implies that counselors are in agreement with its general policies and principles. Counselors strive to reach agreement with employers regarding acceptable standards of client care and professional conduct that allow for changes in institutional policy conducive to the growth and development of clients.

2. **D.1.h. Negative Conditions.** Counselors alert their employers of inappropriate policies and practices. They attempt to effect changes

in such policies or procedures through constructive action within the organization. When such policies are potentially disruptive or damaging to clients or may limit the effectiveness of services provided and change cannot be affected, counselors take appropriate further action. Such action may include referral to appropriate certification, accreditation, or state licensure organizations or voluntary termination of employment.

Applying a Decision-Making Model: Corey, Corey, Corey, and Callanan's Model

1. **Identify the problem or dilemma.** As with any profession, counselors deserve a living wage and benefits to ensure that retirement is feasible. However, the general public seeking supportive services deserves to not have interruptions in treatment that could affect recovery and well-being. Mitzi is currently in the unfortunate position of having to negotiate a conflict between two respective factions within the agency: the employers looking to save money and the employees looking for fair compensation.

2. **Identify the potential issues involved.** While the main concern is Mitzi's role in middle management, her past relationship with Thelma provides an added layer of complexity, as Thelma is clearly struggling to accept Mitzi's new position. Thelma may be acting out of spite, as she may be frustrated with being overlooked for a promotion.

3. **Review the relevant ethics codes.** The ACA Code does not explicitly condone or forbid "unionization," but the actions of T.U.T. are certainly extreme. The code suggests that counselors attempt to effect change through constructive practices, and denying clients services seems to oppose this.

4. **Know the applicable laws and regulations.** One of the main concerns is client abandonment, as the agency runs the risk of denying services to clients if the counselors on staff decide to strike. As such, the agency—and Mitzi in her role as clinical supervisor—need to do everything in their power to avoid having this happen.

5. **Obtain consultation.** Before writing a response to Thelma's email, Mitzi should consult with her direct supervisor regarding agency policies and procedures. One of the details she is likely to encounter is that counselor unionization is likely *not* a viable option for a staff of 10. Unionization works best in organizations with large groups of employees (e.g., Dastagir, 2018). If a staff of this size threatens to quit, it would be relatively easy for the agency to replace them. As such, Mitzi may be in a better position than she realizes.

6. **Consider possible and probable courses of action.** Assuming her supervisors support her position, Mitzi could respond in kind and threaten to allow the staff to quit, delaying treatment for a few weeks as she covers services on her own for emergency cases and hires replacement therapists. She could also refuse to discuss financial concerns directly with supervisees and refer them to the administration at the agency. In either case, Mitzi is not in a position to directly influence the decision made on behalf of the organization.

7. **Enumerate and consider the possible consequences of various decisions.** If Mitzi opts to forward this to the agency's administration, she may miss an opportunity to defuse the situation before things get worse for everyone involved. It may be that allowing Thelma and the other therapists to have their concerns heard and validated would resolve the problem. Also, Mitzi may have the option of managing the agency without the full clinical staff, though she runs the risk of providing substandard care.

8. **Choose what appears to be the best course of action.** Essentially, Thelma and the staff are threatening to harm clients by denying care if their financial needs are not addressed. Mitzi needs to do everything she can to avoid having this happen, but she cannot allow her staff to subject clients to substandard care. The best course of action is likely to try and validate the concerns of the therapists, but to let them know that—unless the agency's administration directs her otherwise—a staff of this size refusing to return to work will simply be let go and replaced.

The Likely Answer

Mitzi should arrange a meeting with Thelma, validate the concerns of all involved in T.U.T., and explain that the company—not her—will let them go if a strike occurs.

ESTABLISHING PROFESSIONAL AND ETHICAL OBLIGATIONS (*FIVE ANGRY COUNSELORS*)

A group of counselors working for a community mental health center are in the middle of weekly supervision. As is customary, one group member presents a case each week to discuss with the group, either as part of a standard rotation or based upon the immediate needs of the group members. This week, E.G. is presenting a case: One of his clients reports to have hit his 6-year-old daughter, and E.G. is uncertain about whether or not he is obligated to file a report with child services.

Upon presenting this case to the group, three of the members are certain that he should file a report. However, two members—E.G. himself and his supervisor, Henry—are of the opinion that he should probably *not* file a report. The majority of the group—three licensed professional counselors with decades of clinical experience among them—believe that this case presents clear evidence of child abuse that requires a direct report to the authorities. However, the minority of the group—the clinician directly responsible for the case and his direct supervisor—are of the opinion that this does *not* constitute abuse.

E.G. wants very much to respect the opinions of his colleagues, but he also wants to abide by his own clinical acumen, and he is supported by his direct supervisor in this decision.

Questions for Discussion

1. *If the majority of his colleagues believe he should report, is E.G. obligated to do so?*
2. *If E.G. does* not *report and the case is eventually found to be evidence of abuse, is Henry liable in any way as his direct supervisor?*
3. *Is there an informal resolution process that can be achieved?*

Straight From the Code

1. **D.1.d. Establishing Professional and Ethical Obligations.** Counselors who are members of interdisciplinary teams work together with team members to clarify professional and ethical obligations of the team as a whole and of its individual members. When a team decision raises ethical concerns, counselors first attempt to resolve the concern within the team. If they cannot reach resolution among team members, counselors pursue other avenues to address their concerns consistent with client well-being.

Applying a Decision-Making Model: Corey, Corey, Corey, and Callanan's Model

1. **Identify the problem or dilemma.** A group of clinicians working for the same organization disagree about the severity of an incident involving a client and the need to report the case to child services. The clinician directly responsible and his direct supervisor are opposed to reporting the incident to child services, but the majority of the group feel otherwise.

2. **Identify the potential issues involved.** It is unclear if *majority rules* applies here in regard to ambiguous ethical decisions or if clinicians are allowed to make their own decision regardless of the opinions of their colleagues. It is also unclear the extent to which liability befalls others at the clinic: Is supervisor Henry directly responsible for the behaviors of his supervisees? Are other members of the team

obligated (or able) to file a report independent of E.G. or Henry as they heard this information indirectly?

3. **Review the relevant ethics codes.** As would be expected, the ACA Code does not directly outline the required course of action. It only states that clinicians work together to identify ethical obligations.

4. **Know the applicable laws and regulations.** Regardless of the Code of Ethics' ambiguity, counselors are mandated reporters where suspicion of child abuse is concerned. A mandated reporter is any individual who may have frequent contact with children, who is required by law to report child maltreatment (National Clearinghouse on Child Abuse and Neglect Information, 2015), with *suspicion* of abuse alone meeting the criteria for a required report. Failure to report an incident of suspected abuse is a serious offense and can result in jail time in some states.

   For E.G., he is obligated to use his best judgment with regard to what constitutes suspicion; however, the same is true of his colleagues. It may be that the group have been respectful of the confidentiality of their clients during these supervisory meetings, as this would likely limit the liability of the members other than E.G. Specifically, if the other group members are unaware of the child's name or identifying information, they would be incapable of filing a report (but could still attempt to do so if they felt strongly enough).

5. **Obtain consultation.** While the nature of this group is consultation, E.G. may benefit from reaching out to his relevant national or state association's ethical advisory committee. While it is unlikely that any advice obtained will provide a definitive answer, the opinion of a third party might help to clarify his thinking, and documented consultation with a professional organization may act as another layer of protection in the event that a complaint is filed with the state licensing board for any reason.

6. **Consider possible and probable courses of action.** Either E.G. can ignore the opinions of his fellow clinicians and move ahead without filing a report (with the support of his direct supervisor), or he can assume that his colleagues see this case more clearly than he does and follow their direction by filing a report.

7. **Enumerate and consider the possible consequences of various decisions.** If E.G. decides *not* to file a report, he is putting himself at risk, but hopefully not also his colleagues (assuming he has only given them basic information regarding client identifying information). However, he retains his ability to act in the best interest of his clients according to his own perspective; if he does not believe—based on all the available information presented—that his client's actions constitute abuse, he is

under no obligation to report (though it could be argued that the opinions of his colleagues may be enough to warrant suspicion). If he *does* decide to file a report, he is erring on the side of caution, though he may also be damaging rapport irreparably with this client.

8. **Choose what appears to be the best course of action.** What constitutes suspicion of abuse is ill defined in most states. If E.G. decides not to file a report, he is putting himself and possibly the child at risk. However, this would be *his* decision, and it is supported by a direct supervisor. Unless there is additional information indicating that this spanking incident falls under the umbrella of abuse in his state, E.G. could trust his opinion and his supervisor's. However, his colleagues are well within their right to file a report of their own if they feel strongly enough about their concerns.

The Likely Answer

The opinions of the majority of the staff in his clinic are that abuse has occurred. Regardless of what E.G. thinks, this is probably enough to warrant *suspicion*, and he should probably file a report.

PERSONNEL SELECTION AND ASSIGNMENT (*WHAT DOES SHE SEE IN HER?*)

Charles is the department chair of a counselor education program at a high-ranking university. Part of his job is to ensure that he has enough faculty on staff to meet the needs of his students as well as the basic requirements to maintain the program's Council for Accreditation of Counseling and Related Educational Programs (CACREP) accreditation. As a faculty member is deciding to retire next year, Charles opens up a search to hire a counselor educator for a tenure-track assistant professor position.

Almost immediately, Charles finds the ideal candidate: Courtney. Courtney is a recent graduate of a CACREP-accredited doctoral program in counselor education. Though she has only held the title *doctor* for less than a month now, her record of scholarship as a graduate student has been phenomenal. Her list of publications and involvement in external grant funding exceeds many of the tenured faculty on staff, her research interests are a perfect fit for the department, and her on-campus interview is described by the search committee as "stellar."

Charles is very aware that Courtney is likely to receive multiple offers, so he works with the dean to put together what he believes will be an enticing package. Courtney counters the offer by agreeing to accept if the university can find a position for her partner: Amanda, a graduate of the same doctoral program as Courtney, with a less impressive record of scholarship overall. Charles argues to the dean that Courtney is their ideal candidate, and they agree to include a nontenure line as a full-time lecturer for Amanda as part of the offer.

Courtney accepts, and her work during the first year is nothing short of exceptional. Amanda, however, is performing poorly. Her teaching evaluations from her first semester are incredibly low, she is rude and confrontational during staff meetings, and several department faculty members have directly complained to Charles that she is damaging the department's reputation. Charles has met with Amanda several times this year to provide feedback and guidance, but her performance seems largely unaffected.

As a new academic year approaches, Charles must decide whether to renew Amanda's contract or not.

Questions for Discussion

1. *Should Charles have hired Courtney and Amanda together? Is hiring a spouse an acceptable part of a job offer for a faculty position?*
2. *Is there a way to remove Amanda from her position without losing Courtney in the process?*
3. *How can Charles make a fair decision in this case without allowing his personal needs (i.e., retaining Courtney) affect his decision-making process?*

Straight From the Code

1. **D.1.f. Personnel Selection and Assignment.** When counselors are in a position requiring personnel selection and/or assigning of responsibilities to others, they select competent staff and assign responsibilities compatible with their skills and experiences.

Applying a Decision-Making Model: Corey, Corey, Corey, and Callanan's Model

1. **Identify the problem or dilemma.** Charles took a risk when he decided to advocate for a spousal hire, and it has now backfired on him completely. Courtney is a valued member of the department with a promising future, whereas Amanda is struggling.

2. **Identify the potential issues involved.** If Charles opts to not renew Amanda's contract, he risks losing Courtney as a faculty member. However, if he decides to bolster the department's connection to Courtney by keeping Amanda on as a faculty member, he is likely doing a disservice to both the students and the other faculty members.

3. **Review the relevant ethics codes.** The ACA Code does not directly outline how to manage a scenario as specific as this. However, it does explicitly state that counselors "select competent staff and assign responsibilities compatible with their skills and experiences." This statement could be taken to mean that if Amanda's behavior is

determined to indicate a lack of competence or skill, Charles would likely be in the right to reassign her to a different position or to simply not renew her contract, regardless of her relationship with Courtney.

4. **Know the applicable laws and regulations.** Depending on the institution, spousal hire situations such as this may occur with some degree of regularity. As an academic dean at Johns Hopkins University, Bell (2010) indicated a third of all faculty recruitment cases during a 3-year period involved negotiations related to spousal hiring. The world of academia as a whole has no specific protocol outlined for managing these negotiations, and the specifics can be complex. Per Bell, deans and department heads have found that in some cases, no amount of practical incentives related to money or other institutional support can convince a person to compromise a relationship with someone they love.

5. **Obtain consultation.** Some of the first places that Charles should look for consultation are the university's policies and procedures manual and the human resources department. Both may be able to provide an overview of specific regulations regarding procedures for hiring and firing, and human resources may be able to provide alternate suggestions beyond simply letting Amanda go (e.g., finding a position for her in the university that does not involve teaching). Charles should also be working directly with his dean to ensure that all decisions are in line with the mission of the university.

6. **Consider possible and probable courses of action.** Depending on what the university, human resources, and his academic dean have to say, Charles is likely to have the option of either working with Amanda to improve her performance overall or to simply let her go.

7. **Enumerate and consider the possible consequences of various decisions.** If Charles decides to not renew Amanda's contract, he runs the risk of losing Courtney, but this may be completely appropriate given the extent to which Amanda has violated the terms of her contract (which likely stipulates that she must maintain a specific level of performance in order to be renewed). However, he has to consider this situation as though Amanda is a completely separate employee (which she is) and remind himself to treat her as an entity completely separate from Courtney. If the university supports denying Amanda a new contract and he opts *not* to let her go after numerous complaints from students and faculty, he is likely not acting in the program's best interest.

8. **Choose what appears to be the best course of action.** Amanda was given a fixed term contract and—despite numerous meetings to address her performance—she has not met its terms. Charles is likely in the right if he decides not to renew her contract, assuming the

university is behind him. He may work with human resources to help find her another position in the university if they are amenable to this, but she has clearly not met the standards necessary to retain her position for another year.

The Likely Answer

Charles needs to be compassionate but firm: Amanda cannot stay on as an instructor.

TEAMWORK AND IMPAIRMENT (*CHECK, PLEASE!*)

Demetri is a counselor working in an outpatient clinic, providing drug and alcohol counseling. He has a close relationship with his coworkers, and they regularly meet for happy hour at the local tavern on Friday evenings. The meetings are typically a low-key affair: He and his colleagues Keith, Steven, and Mario usually have a few beers and talk about pop culture and politics.

On this particular evening, Demetri notices his coworker Keith has had a few too many drinks. While Demetri and the rest of the crew are all at their usual table, Keith has said that he needs to "blow off a little steam" and is talking to some younger women near the end of the bar. He is slurring his speech and making quite a spectacle of himself.

Worse yet, Demetri overhears him sharing a personal anecdote from a group counseling session that Keith ran earlier today. Keith even goes so far as to refer to the client in his story by name.

Questions for Discussion

1. *Should Demetri do anything to intervene in the moment, or should he just wait until Keith sobers up?*
2. *Should Demetri report this incident to Keith's direct supervisor?*
3. *Is anyone obligated to inform the client about this potential breach of confidentiality?*

Straight From the Code

1. **C.2.g. Impairment.** Counselors monitor themselves for signs of impairment from their own physical, mental, or emotional problems and refrain from offering or providing professional services when impaired. They seek assistance for problems that reach the level of professional impairment, and, if necessary, they limit, suspend, or terminate their professional responsibilities until it is determined that they may safely resume their work. Counselors assist colleagues or supervisors in recognizing their own professional impairment and provide consultation and assistance when warranted with colleagues

or supervisors showing signs of impairment and intervene as appropriate to prevent imminent harm to clients.

2. **D.1.c. Interdisciplinary Teamwork.** Counselors who are members of interdisciplinary teams delivering multifaceted services to clients remain focused on how to best serve clients. They participate in and contribute to decisions that affect the well-being of clients by drawing on the perspectives, values, and experiences of the counseling profession and those of colleagues from other disciplines.

Applying a Decision-Making Model: Corey, Corey, Corey, and Callanan's Model

1. **Identify the problem or dilemma.** This one is pretty straightforward: Keith is drunk and sharing personal information about his clients with the other bar patrons.

2. **Identify the potential issues involved.** In this setting, Demetri is in no way directly responsible for his colleague's behavior. If Keith is removed from the bar for being intoxicated, this is not Demetri's responsibility. However, Keith *is* behaving in such a way that the clients at Demetri's place of employment are potentially being harmed.

3. **Review the relevant ethics codes.** The ACA Code is surprisingly clear in cases such as this: Counselors assist colleagues or supervisors in recognizing their own professional impairment and provide consultation and assistance when warranted, and they remain focused on how to best serve clients. However, the expectation is that counselors will attempt to resolve areas of conflict among themselves first before escalating the concern to a licensing board or supervisor (I.2.a.).

4. **Know the applicable laws and regulations.** Criminal proceedings regarding breaches of confidentiality are unlikely, but a client who has been betrayed in this way may be well within his or her right to file a complaint with a licensing board or a civil suit (Soeiro, 2018). In this case, however, the client is completely unaware that a breach has occurred, and Demetri may well be the only individual aware of the extent to which Keith has betrayed his client's trust. In short, it is likely that no criminal law has been broken here, but Demetri should feel a strong moral obligation.

5. **Obtain consultation.** Demetri's only option for consultation (apart from googling the ACA Code of Ethics and state law regarding confidentiality on his cell phone) is to make his other colleagues aware of what Keith is doing and discuss how best to proceed.

6. **Consider possible and probable courses of action.** Given the code's wording, it seems unlikely that Demetri can ignore what has happened.

One option would be to intervene immediately, with Demetri confronting Keith in the moment and admonishing his behavior. Another option would be for Keith to address the incident later, specifically at a time when Keith is sober and lucid.

7. **Enumerate and consider the possible consequences of various decisions.** If Demetri intervenes in the moment, Keith may respond with an apology, or he may respond with anger. However, not preventing Keith from further disclosures in the moment may put clients at additional risk.

8. **Choose what appears to be the best course of action.** Demetri should likely begin by addressing Keith directly, but privately, and appeal to his sensibilities as a clinician in doing so. Regardless of whether Demetri addresses Keith in the moment, Demetri should also plan to meet with Keith at a later date when he is sober to discuss the incident in more explicit detail and offer support in addition to expressing concern. If Keith refuses to accept responsibility for this incident, it might be acceptable to have a discussion about what occurred with his direct supervisor as well.

The Likely Answer

Demetri needs to pull Keith aside in the moment, talk with him again the next day, and bring it up with the rest of the group and relevant administrative staff if he feels the problem has not been effectively resolved.

CONFIDENTIALITY IN THE WORKPLACE (*YOU KNOW WHAT I MEAN*)

Gina is a counselor working in an inpatient hospital setting. As part of her daily lunch routine, she goes into the staff lounge to heat up her tomato soup and get a coffee.

Today, when she walks into the staff lounge to begin her soup preparation, she hears two social workers talking about one of the clients that Gina admitted and has been seeing for family therapy: 12-year-old Emily who has a history of trauma and repeated suicide attempts. Gina immediately recognizes that they are talking about Emily, as one of them makes a disparaging remark about Emily's recent suicide attempt and her behavior with other children on the unit.

Tomato soup in hand, Gina freezes as one of the social workers says to the other, "Emily is a liar and is always just trying to get attention." The other social worker then turns to Gina and says, "You know what we mean, Gina. You see her for individual counseling, right?"

Gina looks down at her lunch and is unsure of how to respond. She smiles awkwardly, shakes her head, and tries to change the subject to how long it takes to heat up soup. After heating up her lunch, she leaves to eat in the hospital cafeteria to avoid any additional conversation about Emily. She feels unsettled by these comments and is unsure how to respond.

Questions for Discussion

1. *Is the staff lounge a secure enough space for a conversation about a client?*
2. *Whose code of ethics applies to this discussion: the National Association of Social Workers or the American Counseling Association?*
3. *Should Gina report this behavior to a supervisor or just ignore that it happened?*

Straight From the Code

1. **D.1.b. Forming Relationships.** Counselors work to develop and strengthen relationships with colleagues from other disciplines to best serve clients.

2. **D.1.d. Establishing Professional and Ethical Obligations.** Counselors who are members of interdisciplinary teams work together with team members to clarify professional and ethical obligations of the team as a whole and of its individual members. When a team decision raises ethical concerns, counselors first attempt to resolve the concern within the team. If they cannot reach resolution among team members, counselors pursue other avenues to address their concerns consistent with client well-being.

Applying a Decision-Making Model: Corey, Corey, Corey, and Callanan's Model

1. **Identify the problem or dilemma.** Gina's colleagues are discussing one of her clients in a location that is on site (i.e., within the hospital), but one that is in no way identified as a secure space. Their intentions do not seem outwardly malicious, in that her colleagues want to vent their frustrations with other coworkers and are inviting Gina to join in on the conversation. It could be argued that this may potentially help the coworkers (and Gina) strengthen their workplace relationships (D.1.b.). However, limits of confidentiality dictate what they are allowed to discuss. The problem lies in whether the staff lounge is a place to have confidential conversations, and if Gina should take part in this exchange.

2. **Identify the potential issues involved.** Since it is a conversation in a potentially public space outside of normal working hours (e.g., a lunch break), it does not fall under the umbrella of supervision, but it could be defined as consultation. However, the space is not identified

as a secure location where others—whether they are other colleagues not involved in the conversation or other clients near or outside of the staff lounge—would be unable to hear what is being discussed.

However, Gina could compromise her relationship with her colleagues by choosing not to join in on the conversation. Reporting them to a supervisor would likely betray their trust as well.

3. **Review the relevant ethics codes.** While not a part of section D, the ACA Code of Ethics requires adherence to confidentiality with some exceptions for supervision and consultation (B.7.a.). However, section D makes it clear that a misstep regarding ethics needs to be addressed by the team (D.1.d.), regardless of the team member's affiliation as a social worker. As such, Gina may need to inform her colleagues of their oversight: Specifically, that the parameters of confidentiality are to be followed, unless seeking consultation.

   On the other hand, it is also prevalent in the Code to maintain positive working relationships with other counselors. This means that Gina needs to find a way to present her concerns to her peers in a way that does not damage their working relationship.

4. **Know the applicable laws and regulations.** Gina should be well versed in her hospital's institutional policies and procedures, as privacy law is likely to be an influencing factor. The Health Insurance Portability and Accountability Act of 1996 prohibits the sharing of confidential client information and financial penalties can be imposed. Discussion of clients outside of supervision directly violates the codes of confidentiality set forth by the ACA ethical code as well as HIPAA.

5. **Obtain consultation.** While there are no additional colleagues or supervisors for her to consult in this moment, Gina could bring up the issue in supervision and ask her supervisor what the best course of action would be in this scenario.

6. **Consider possible and probable courses of action.** Gina could join in and discuss the client, as well as relate to her coworkers, which would likely strengthen their relationship (albeit at the potential expense of a client's confidence). She could also inform her colleagues of the inappropriate and unethical conversation they are having and help them understand the limits of what they can and cannot discuss in a public space. However, this would likely cause some amount of disruption in Gina's relationship with her peers.

7. **Enumerate and consider the possible consequences of various decisions.** If Gina decides to join the conversation, she may be directly violating HIPAA regulations and the ACA Code of Ethics. On the other hand, if she does not join, Gina is missing a possible chance to strengthen her relationship with these coworkers.

8. **Choose what appears to be the best course of action.** Ultimately, it is more important for Gina to meet the needs of her clients. The trick in this case would be finding a way to initiate a conversation with her coworkers in such a way that does not betray her coworkers' confidence as well.

The Likely Answer

Gina could join the conversation, but only to inform her colleagues (gently, politely, and with empathy) about the importance of confidentiality as per the ACA Code of Ethics.

PROTECTION FROM PUNITIVE ACTION (*THIS PLACE IS MAKING ME SICK*)

Brittany is a counselor in a community mental health facility. She has been getting sick for the past 3 months after her office was moved to another floor. Despite her best efforts at managing her symptoms with vitamins and ibuprofen, she keeps coming down with sinus infections and has started to miss work once or twice a week for the past month and a half.

After conversing with three other counselors, Brittany learns that they too have been experiencing the same symptoms since they moved to this floor. The other employees have not endured as many sinus issues, and they have been coming to work regularly; however, they did report taking off at least 1 day in the past month and a half.

The staff clinical supervisor has told Brittany and the other employees that this is "all in their heads and nothing is wrong with the office." Brittany reported her medical issues and the comment from the supervisor to the facility director. The facility director said the matter would be looked into but also indicated the belief that this was "much ado about nothing."

Brittany waited a week to follow up and reported this to the Occupational Safety and Health Administration (OSHA). Her supervisor was made aware of this and informed all staff that OSHA would be coming in and that all employees were "not to say anything to them."

Almost immediately after the OSHA visit was scheduled, Brittany was notified by her supervisor that she was being placed on administrative leave. The supervisor said the reason for this administrative leave was due to Brittany "not being at her post," which means not reporting to work regularly and taking too many sick days in a short period of time.

Questions for Discussion

1. *Should Brittany have been put on administrative leave for missing work due to illness?*
2. *Should Brittany attempt to resolve this directly with her supervisor?*
3. *Can/should the counselor file a complaint about the supervisor? If so, whom does she file it with?*

Straight From the Code

D.1.i. Protection From Punitive Action. Counselors do not harass a colleague or employee or dismiss an employee who has acted in a responsible and ethical manner to expose inappropriate employer policies or practices.

Applying a Decision-Making Model: Corey, Corey, Corey, and Callanan's Model

1. **Identify the problem or dilemma.** Brittany was well within her right to report the health and safety concerns at her place of employment. Despite her supervisor's frustrations with the outcome, they likely acted unethically by placing her on administrative leave (unless it can be determined that Brittany's behavior is part of a longstanding pattern). The question at this point is: How should Brittany respond?

2. **Identify the potential issues involved.** Being placed on administrative leave causes several concerns for Brittany's well-being, with regard to both her mental health and financial security. The real reason for her administrative leave may actually be that the administration of Brittany's place of employment does not want her present during OSHA's investigation of the facility. Additionally, Brittany may have been unable to terminate with clients or set up plans for transition, therefore creating a concern for continuity of care for each client.

   However, it should be noted once again that this case only presents one side of the story. If Brittany has a history of missing work or regular conflicts with her supervisor, her supervisor's decision may have been appropriate.

3. **Review the relevant ethics codes.** The ACA Code clearly states that counselors should be capable of reporting workplace concerns without fear of retribution. Assuming Brittany does not have a longstanding history of work-related difficulties, it is reasonable to assume that her supervisor may have acted unethically.

4. **Know the applicable laws and regulations.** OSHA indicates that under their "whistle-blower" laws, an employee cannot be harmed for reporting unsafe working conditions. There is also the right of refusal to work in any case where an individual is exposed to potential harm. In this case, the staff is protected under federal law if they choose to report.

   In this instance, it may be helpful for Brittany to review how complaints are filed in the organization, and what the process is. She may also want to know if she is still to be compensated, if she can continue receiving insurance benefits, and how this impacts a return to employment. She should also refer to specific laws regarding employment in her state.

5. **Obtain consultation.** Brittany might want to consult with legal counsel, a union representative (if applicable), other coworkers, and/or medical professionals. As a member of the ACA, she might also set up a consultation call with the ACA ethics committee.

6. **Consider possible and probable courses of action.** Brittany could decide if it is worth pursuing a legal path against her employer, or she could ask to have a meeting with her supervisor and director to understand more about the administrative leave. She could also complete the leave, return to work, and put the incident behind her and act as if nothing happened.

7. **Enumerate and consider the possible consequences of various decisions.** It might be easy to just ignore the placement on administrative leave; however, it will likely be challenging to come back to her previous clients and explain why she was gone for a period of time. It might also change the workplace culture, since she will not be present when OSHA does their site visit. If she decides to pursue legal action and returns after the leave, it might or might not create a hostile work environment. If at some point she decides to leave the setting, she might need to explain to her next employer why she was placed on administrative leave, and she may be unable to obtain support or a recommendation from the previous employer.

8. **Choose what appears to be the best course of action.** Brittany should first decide what constitutes a reasonable outcome in this situation: Would it be to have the administrative leave removed? Is it the opportunity to speak with OSHA directly?

   Whatever her needs may be, the most reasonable course of action for Brittany is likely to begin by reaching out to her supervisor's supervisor. If this does not provide her with a reasonable outcome, she may consider reaching out to legal counsel if applicable. Additionally, it would be in her best interest to document (or obtain documentation of) any and all interactions prior to the leave.

The Likely Answer

Brittany should decide what she needs to feel that a resolution has been achieved. She should then attempt to contact her supervisor's supervisor. If she is still left feeling that justice has not occurred, she could reach out to a lawyer.

IN-CLASS DISCUSSION AND EXERCISES

Group Discussion: Recognizing Potential Tripping Points (Coworkers)

Think about your own work history and your potential *tripping points* related to interactions with colleagues. Who have been the coworkers that you got along with? Who were the ones you struggled with? Have there been specific personalities that triggered you in some way? Have there been specific work-related concerns that caused you to get upset more easily than others?

Group Discussion: Difficult Conversations (Coworkers)

A hallmark of the cases in this section is the idea that some conversations can be both challenging and uncomfortable. Confronting coworkers or other professionals is never enjoyable, and devising practical methods for doing so can get pretty abstract.

Imagine you had to confront one of your colleagues for drinking too much at a work function. How would you go about this? What would you do to prepare for this conversation? Is there anything practical that you could do in advance of this discussion? Are you the type who prepares a script beforehand? Do you do better with improvisation? Are there specific colleagues that you would have an easier time doing this with? Why?

Role Play: Counselors Unite!

Using the scenario described in *Counselors Unite!*, role-play possible outcomes. Have one member play the role of Mitzi and another play the role of Thelma discussing the situation at hand. If you were Mitzi, how might you begin a dialogue? As Thelma, how might you actually feel or respond in the moment if Mitzi were to make efforts at resolving this matter directly?

Documentation: Problem, Data, Assessment, and Plan

Using the Problem, Data, Assessment, and Plan (PDAP) format, pick one of the cases and write a progress note indicating the following:

Problem: What were the presenting concerns of this particular interaction?

Data: What, objectively, has happened? Remember to write this without subjective language or interpretation.

Assessment: As the counselor or supervisor in question, what *should* be done? Be sure to demonstrate comprehensive use of the decision-making model in this section.

Plan: What *will* be done? Be sure to outline a comprehensive plan that relates to the decision-making model.

References

Bell, D. A. (2010). The intricacies of spousal hiring. *The Chronicle of Higher Education*. Retrieved from https://www.chronicle.com/article/The-Intricacies-of-Spousal/65456

Corey, G., Corey, M. S., Corey, C., & Callanan, P. (2015). *Issues and ethics in the helping professions* (9th ed.). Stamford, CT: Brooks/Cole.

Council on Social Work Education. (2015). *Council on Social Work Education Educational Policy and Accreditation Standards*. Washington, DC: CSWE.

Dastagir, A. E. (2018). Will your therapist go on strike? 4,000 mental health workers protest Kaiser Permanente. *USA Today*. Retrieved from https://www.usatoday.com/story/news/nation/2018/12/07/kaiser-permanente-strike-mental-health-workers-california-therapists/2225472002/

Jacob, C. J. (2013). Domestic violence and couples counseling: The importance of assessment and understanding typologies in treatment. *Journal of Family Psychotherapy, 24*(4), 286–295. doi:10.1080/08975353.2013.849553

National Association of Social Workers. (2017). *National Association of Social Workers Code of Ethics*. Washington, DC: NASW.

National Clearinghouse on Child Abuse and Neglect Information. (2015). *Mandatory reporters of child abuse and neglect*. Retrieved from https://www.childwelfare.gov/pubPDFs/manda.pdf

Soeiro, L. (2018). My therapist shared my secrets, and other horror stories: When therapists can't keep their patients' private information to themselves. *Psychology Today*. Retrieved from https://www.psychologytoday.com/us/blog/i-hear-you/201803/my-therapist-shared-my-secrets-and-other-horror-stories

CHAPTER 5

EVALUATION, ASSESSMENT, AND INTERPRETATION (SECTION E OF THE ACA CODE OF ETHICS)

INTRODUCTION

Counseling's relationship with testing and assessment is at times convoluted; and while assessment remains an important aspect of counseling, testing and evaluation are often relegated to psychology. Though wellness-oriented approaches are often at odds with the labels inherent in these practices, counselors are often required to make use of tests and evaluations either as a component of their own practice or to coordinate care with insurance providers or other clinicians. The scenarios in this section highlight the ways in which assessment in general can become a complex area of practice.

All cases will be assessed using Garcia, Cartwright, Winston, and Borzuchowska's (2003) Transcultural Integrative Model for making an ethical decision.

GARCIA, CARTWRIGHT, WINSTON, AND BORZUCHOWSKA'S TRANSCULTURAL INTEGRATIVE MODEL

The transcultural integrative model by Garcia, Cartwright, Winston, and Borzuchowska (2003) makes culture the central concept in the ethical decision-making process. This model offers counselors the structure of a linear, step-by-step model. However, it also incorporates collaborative and social constructivist concepts requiring a great deal of reflection, collaboration, and consensus seeking. The model contains four steps:

1. **Interpreting the situation through awareness and fact finding.**

    a. **This model requires an enhancement of sensitivity and awareness.** Counselors must consider the emotions, needs, and general welfare of all involved, including themselves. The first step in the process involves both an exploration of what is known and an internal assessment of what the counselor knows (and does not know).

    b. **Specific areas of consideration include but are not limited to the following:** who are the major stakeholders; counselor attitudes and emotional reactions toward cultural groups; counselor knowledge of client's culture; counselor awareness of cultural identity, acculturation, and role socialization of self and client; counselor awareness of own multicultural counseling competence skills; whether a dilemma has occurred; and what are the relevant cultural considerations.

2. **Formulating an ethical decision.** Counselors review the dilemma (if there is one) and determine whether the dilemma has changed or not in light of the new information gathered in step 1.

   a. **Specific areas of consideration include but are not limited to the following:** determine relevant ethical codes, laws, ethical principles, institution policies, and procedures; determine the ethics laws and practice applicable to the situation; examine potential discriminatory laws, institutional policies, and procedures; estimate potential conflict between laws and ethics resulting from a cultural perspective.

   b. **Generate courses of action.** As a component of step 2, counselors list all possible and probable courses of action. Make sure the courses of action selected reflect the cultural worldview of the parties involved. Use relational method and social constructivism techniques (negotiating, working toward consensus, and arbitrating) as appropriate to reach agreement on potential courses of action.

   c. **Consider potential positive and negative consequences for each course of action.** Counselors then list both positive and negative consequences under each of the courses of action selected. Consider the positive and negative consequences of each course of action from within the cultural worldview of each of the parties involved. Again, consider using a relational method and social constructivism techniques to reach agreement on analyzing consequences.

   d. **Consultation.** Counselors then consult with supervisors and other knowledgeable professionals, particularly those who have pertinent multicultural expertise.

   e. **Select the best ethical course of action.** Based on a rational analysis of the consequences and ethical principles underlying the competing courses of action, counselors determine the best course of action. This decision should best represent an agreement between the cultural worldview of the client and that of the other parties involved. Use social constructivism techniques to choose a course of action that is mutually satisfying to key parties.

3. **Weighing competing, nonmoral values and affirming the course of action.**

   a. **Engage in reflective recognition and analysis of personal blind spots.** Counselors identify nonmoral values that may interfere with the implementation of the course of action selected, particularly those values that may be reflecting a culture different from the client's culture.

b. **Consider contextual influences on values selection.** Counselors consider the contextual influences on values selection at the collegial, professional team, institutional, cultural, and societal levels.

4. **Planning and executing the selected course of action.**

   a. **Develop a reasonable sequence of concrete actions.** Counselors divide the course of action into simple, sequential actions. They identify culturally relevant resources and strategies for the implementation of the plan.

   b. **Anticipate personal and contextual barriers and countermeasures.** Anticipate and confront personal and contextual barriers to the successful implementation of the plan of action and take appropriate countermeasures. Counselors should again be aware of cultural barriers such as biases, discrimination, stereotypes, and prejudices and develop effective and relevant culture-specific countermeasures.

   c. **Implementation, documentation, and evaluation of the course of action.** Finally, the course of action is executed as planned. It is recommended to document valid and reliable information and evaluate the accuracy of the course of action in its aftermath. Use a relational method and social constructivism techniques to identify measures and data sources that include both universal and culture-specific variables.

The expansion of the integrative model to include a multicultural component reflects the authors' recognition of the increasing importance of cultural context, intersectionality, and the (hopefully) expanding demographic of clients accessing counseling services.

LIMITS OF COMPETENCE (*DON'T TEST ME…*)

Rocky is a second-year counseling student at a Council for Accreditation of Counseling and Related Educational Programs (CACREP)–accredited counselor training program, with a focus on clinical mental health. He was fortunate enough to land an internship with Mick, a dually licensed counselor and psychologist in charge of a community mental health clinic near campus. The site is an ideal fit for Rocky as he hopes to one day manage a clinic of his own.

As the internship's first semester progresses, however, Rocky begins to feel a bit disillusioned. He finds that very little of his time spent under Mick's supervision is focused on direct client work, as he is instead saddled with administrative duties related to the clinic's operations. Most days, Rocky runs a group in the afternoon but spends most of the morning submitting insurance claims and other billing concerns related to the practice's day-to-day operations.

This week, Mick has asked Rocky to start helping out by writing score reports for some of the Wechsler Adult Intelligence Scale-IV (WAIS-IV) tests that Mick has been administering to clients.

Questions for Discussion

1. *As a counseling intern, is Rocky qualified to score or interpret intelligence tests that have been administered by a licensed psychologist?*
2. *Is testing and assessment a part of the counseling profession?*
3. *Regardless of whether scoring IQ tests is appropriate, is there anything Rocky should do to address his concerns about the nature of his training overall?*

Straight From the Code

1. **E.2.a. Limits of Competence.** Counselors use only those testing and assessment services for which they have been trained and are competent. Counselors using technology-assisted test interpretations are trained in the construct being measured and the specific instrument being used prior to using its technology-based application. Counselors take reasonable measures to ensure the proper use of assessment techniques by persons under their supervision.

Applying a Decision-Making Model: Garcia, Cartwright, Winston, and Borzuchowska's Transcultural Integrative Model

1. **Interpreting the situation through awareness and fact finding.** An important component of the model of Garcia, Cartwright, Winston, and Borzuchowska (2003) is recognizing the influence of context and environment in making ethical decisions. Though this case initially focuses on the quality of Rocky's training experience, it would be important to consider the populations served by Mick's clinic and the extent to which clients are being exploited by any of the clinic's practices. For example, the misuse of intelligence testing has a storied history in the profession of psychology (e.g., Kincheloe, Steinberg, & Gresson, 1997), and the clinic's work with marginalized populations should be considered.

2. **Formulating an ethical decision.** In addition to examining the clinic's impact on marginalized populations, it would also be important to consider Mick's adherence to the American Psychological Association (APA) Code of Ethics. Per the APA code, "Psychologists do not promote the use of psychological assessment techniques by unqualified persons, except when such use is conducted for training purposes with appropriate supervision" (9.07, 2010). In this case, Mick may be acting outside the boundaries of his profession's ethics, as he is training Rocky as a counselor, not as a psychologist.

   If Mick has provided Rocky with adequate training such that he understands the nuances of scoring the WAIS-IV well enough to ensure its accurate use, Mick's actions may be appropriate. However, this exam is delegated to licensed psychologists, and its administration and interpretation are complex (see Weiss, Saklofske, Coalson, & Raiford, 2010 for a detailed review). As his training is in counseling, it is unlikely that Rocky is competent enough to administer or score this exam on his own.

3. **Weighing competing, nonmoral values and affirming the course of action.** It seems unlikely that Rocky could ignore these events, as they have a direct impact on his training and the clients he serves. Having a counseling student intern score an exam that could potentially affect a person's life trajectory is likely inappropriate, particularly if the clients being served represent marginalized populations. As such, Rocky will likely have to address the situation with Mick either directly or by proxy through his university.

   As Rocky is a subordinate to Mick, he may feel uncomfortable addressing him directly. However, if Rocky addresses the issue with his internship supervisor at the university first, this will likely create some amount of anxiety for Mick.

4. **Planning and executing the selected course of action.** As there exists a potential for harm to clients, Rocky has to address the issue, but it may be best for him to ask his university supervisor to initiate the process. In doing so, Rocky could potentially maintain rapport with Mick if his internship at this site is salvageable, as the incident could be framed as a concern brought up by the university based on Rocky's report of internship activities (as opposed to Rocky making complaints about his direct supervisor). A direct complaint to any licensing board is likely inappropriate at this time, as the American Counseling Association (ACA) Code of Ethics promotes informal resolutions before filing a report (I.2.a.).

The Likely Answer

Rocky should refrain from writing any score reports and speak directly to his advisor at his academic institution about his concerns.

PREJUDICE IN DIAGNOSIS OF PATHOLOGY (*SUPERVISORS NEED SUPERVISION*)

KatieJane is a recent graduate of a counselor education program. She is currently completing her supervised hours at an outpatient drug and alcohol treatment center where she sees individuals for group and individual treatment as part of an intensive outpatient program. Her supervisor Crispin is a graduate of the same program, albeit 20 years before

KatieJane was born (she is in her 20s, and he is in his 70s). Overall, KatieJane enjoys her weekly supervision meetings with Crispin, and she has been grateful both to find a site with a licensed professional counselor to provide supervision and to have a supervisor with such extensive experience.

This week, KatieJane has met a new client, Belinda, for the first time. Belinda identifies as a trans woman, and KatieJane asks Crispin if they can spend some of their time in supervision this week discussing her case. Specifically, KatieJane has never worked with a trans-identified client before, and she would like some guidance to make sure she is providing support that is sensitive and affirming to both her client's experiences and identity.

KatieJane brings this up in weekly supervision. In response to this request, Crispin rolls his eyes and says, "If you ask me, the whole 'trans thing' seems a little overboard these days." He goes on to say that he does not agree with the idea that gender is both fluid and an innate construct and that he worries about the impact that these ideas have on young children.

Supervision begins to feel very awkward for KatieJane following this exchange, as Crispin's reported personal values are not in keeping with her training.

Questions for Discussion

1. *If Crispin's values are not in keeping with the counseling profession, is he able to practice as a counselor? Is it acceptable to simply disagree with the values of his profession if it does not cause direct harm to clients?*
2. *If KatieJane feels uncomfortable with Crispin's values, can she continue with him as a supervisor?*
3. *Regardless of the long-term concerns about this exchange, what should KatieJane do or say in the moment?*

Straight From the Code

1. **E.5.b. Cultural Sensitivity.** Counselors recognize that culture affects the manner in which clients' problems are defined and experienced. Clients' socioeconomic and cultural experiences are considered when diagnosing mental disorders.

2. **E.5.c. Historical and Social Prejudices in the Diagnosis of Pathology.** Counselors recognize historical and social prejudices in the misdiagnosis and pathologizing of certain individuals and groups and strive to become aware of and address such biases in themselves or others.

Applying a Decision-Making Model: Garcia, Cartwright, Winston, and Borzuchowska's Transcultural Integrative Model

1. **Interpreting the situation through awareness and fact finding.** Though this case initially focuses on the ethics of supervision and supervisor values, the impact this has on clients served by the clinic needs to be considered. One of the major changes to the ACA Code of Ethics in 2014 relates to counselors' responsibilities when making client referrals; specifically, counselors may not refer out clients on the basis of their own discomfort, as this is likely to cause harm to clients (Kaplan et al., 2017). The concern in this case is the impact of Crispin's values on both KatieJane as his supervisee and the clients they are treating. Much has been made of this change in the standards of the ACA Code, with recent legal cases setting the precedent that counselors may not impose personal values that have a detrimental impact on the clients they serve (Hutchens, Block, & Young, 2013).

   However, it should be noted in this case that Crispin has made no actions that are directly harming clients. He has in no way indicated that he intends to discriminate against clients as a function of their identity, and he has not directed KatieJane to do so either. He has simply expressed his personal beliefs in a professional setting.

2. **Formulating an ethical decision.** KatieJane is in a difficult position, as the code clearly advocates for sensitivity in assigning labels of any kind, but Crispin's actions seem more in keeping with the opposite: He is *refusing* to recognize a diagnostic label, and he is negating the historical and social prejudices faced by the trans-identified population. His inability to recognize the validity of trans identities is likely not in keeping with the basic values of the counseling profession.

   However, it should again be noted that Crispin's disclosure is not necessarily an indication of a belief that guides his practice. He did not discuss his efforts to withhold treatment by way of withholding a diagnosis, and he has indicated nothing other than a belief. If KatieJane's concern is whether his admission of a personal value is a direct contradiction to the code of ethics in a way that directly affects his clients, there is little information to go on at this time.

3. **Weighing competing, nonmoral values and affirming the course of action.** It seems unlikely that KatieJane should ignore this comment, though her options are to either address this in the moment with Crispin or escalate the concern to a supervisor above him. As in the previous case, escalating this to a higher level may be inappropriate as the ACA Code promotes informal resolutions before filing a report (I.2.a.). However, KatieJane as a subordinate would have to essentially reprimand a supervisor, which would put her in an awkward position to say the very least.

If the goal is to ensure that the clients treated by the clinic are not being harmed, KatieJane has an obligation to follow up with further inquiry of some kind. It is not her obligation to make direct efforts at challenging Crispin's beliefs (and to be clear: He is in his own right to have them), but Garcia's model is in keeping with the ideas of social justice. Specifically, while counselors are not tasked with policing morality or individual belief, they are ideally acting as advocates for the well-being of all clients.

4. **Planning and executing the selected course of action.** One place for KatieJane to start would be to simply follow up this statement with further inquiry: When Crispin indicated his struggles in believing the existence of the trans identity, was he saying that he does not treat these individuals in his practice, that this makes his practice difficult as it requires him to adapt his work around a personal belief, or that he is imposing his own values on his clients in his practice? Is he suggesting that KatieJane, as a counselor at the clinic, negate Belinda's gender identity?

   However, if KatieJane feels that her work or position would be compromised by expounding on this discussion, it would likely be appropriate to discuss the matter with Crispin's supervisor or no one at all. KatieJane should *not* have to feel as though her position may be compromised in some way by challenging her supervisor directly or indirectly, particularly as there is no evidence that any clients are being harmed at this time (again, Crispin only expressed a personal belief in a professional setting). Unfortunately, none of these options is ideal, as they, respectively, risk damaging her relationship with Crispin, condemning him for his belief by involving a supervisor, or potentially risk the likelihood that clients are being marginalized by a counselor in a position of authority.

   If KatieJane opts not to confront Crispin, however, the quality of her supervision is in question. While it is true that Crispin only stated a personal belief, he expressed this belief in a professional setting with one of his supervisees.

The Likely Answer

KatieJane has the option of asking Crispin what he meant, requesting that his supervisor ask him the same question, and presenting her concerns to the center if she feels she is not receiving adequate supervision or if she believes the welfare of her clients is being compromised in some way.

PROPER DIAGNOSIS (*LIES, LIES, LIES*)

Jaco is a recently licensed counselor working in private practice. He is paneled with an insurance company in the area, and he finds that this has been a relatively easy way to secure a regular base of steady clients. Business overall is going well, though his profit margins tend to be pretty thin from month to month given the price of rent in the area where he practices.

One of his clients, Victor, has been seeing him steadily for several weeks to address anxiety in the aftermath of his divorce. Jaco had been billing under a diagnosis of *adjustment disorder with anxiety* as his symptoms were problematic but not severe enough to meet criteria for anything other than adjustment. This month, however, the insurance company has denied Jaco's claims, stating that they will no longer be paying claims related to adjustment disorders alone.

Victor is a member of the Cherokee nation (a marginalized population in Jaco's area of practice) and has had money troubles in the aftermath of his divorce. Jaco knows that Victor cannot afford his full fee, but he also knows that he cannot afford to allow for sliding scale payments at this time.

He is also aware that Victor's insurance company *will* pay a claim for posttraumatic stress disorder (PTSD) and that Victor could technically meet these criteria if the documentation is submitted correctly.

Questions for Discussion

1. *Is it acceptable to adjust a diagnosis to aid a client in need of assistance?*
2. *If the chances of repercussion are low and the benefits to Victor are potentially high, is it justified to falsify an insurance claim?*
3. *Since the nature of diagnostic impressions is subjective to begin with, could it even be argued that Victor is wrong in the case of either diagnosis? Is diagnosis an arbitrary construct where counseling is concerned?*

Straight From the Code

1. **E.5.a. Proper Diagnosis.** Counselors take special care to provide proper diagnosis of mental disorders. Assessment techniques (including personal interviews) used to determine client care (e.g., locus of treatment, type of treatment, recommended follow-up) are carefully selected and appropriately used.

Applying a Decision-Making Model: Garcia, Cartwright, Winston, and Borzuchowska's Transcultural Integrative Model

1. **Interpreting the situation through awareness and fact finding.** As is the case for all situations examined through the lens of Garcia et al., it is important to examine the impact that decisions have on clients and client values. In this case, Victor is part of a marginalized group, and he may be unable to continue with treatment if Jaco is unable

to accommodate him. Additionally, bias within diagnosis has been established as a significant problem for decades now (e.g., Becker & Lamb, 1994; Woodward, Taft, Gordon, & Meis, 2009), with some arguing its relevance as a construct in professional counseling should be called into question (Bonino & Hanna, 2018).

Still, insurance fraud is a crime and one that could result in prison if it were to be proven in court that Jaco lied to an insurance company to procure additional funding of any kind, regardless of the benefits or detriments to the client. The element of temptation for Jaco in this case may be that diagnosis is essentially an abstract concept. Specifically, a surgeon lying to an insurance company about the extent of a patient's physical injury to procure additional funding may be easily determined as false (e.g., a bone is either broken or not). In the case of a counselor arguing the severity of mental suffering, the elusive nature of psychological distress would make it difficult to determine the accuracy of any claim.

2. **Formulating an ethical decision.** Despite these ideas, the code is very clear in its stance on the matter: Counselors take special care to provide *proper* diagnosis. This suggests that a counselor weighs all of the relevant facts, uses appropriate assessment techniques, and provides an accurate diagnosis no matter the circumstances. In this case, it is assumed that Jaco did all of this in the initial stages of treatment.

3. **Weighing competing, nonmoral values and affirming the course of action.** ...or did he? Jaco may be within his right to reexamine the initial diagnosis at this time by reconsidering the presenting symptoms and their severity. Did he thoroughly rule out a diagnosis of PTSD? Are there assessment instruments he did not consider?

   The obvious problem in reexamining this assessment boils down to a quote attributed to Maslow: If all you have is a hammer, then all you see are nails. In this case, Jaco would have to take special care to ensure that his reassessment is more accurate (rather than less). As such, he should likely work with a supervisor or colleague to review any new assessments he attempts to offer.

   Another option would simply be to accept his initial assessment as accurate. This may be a sensible option, as his current efforts are influenced by a specific need, whereas his initial assessment was likely not influenced by any specific bias related to client needs. Assuming this is the case, he will need to provide Victor with reasonable alternative care options, such as clinicians who will work with him on a sliding scale or local community mental health clinics.

4. **Planning and executing the selected course of action.** If Jaco decides to abide by his decision, he will have to work closely with Victor to ensure that his care is continued. If he decides instead to reassess his

current diagnosis, he will have to make certain that he first uses unbiased assessment techniques in doing so. For example, if he genuinely feels that PTSD may be a presenting concern, he might make use of a standardized instrument such as the PTSD Checklist (Ruggiero, Del Ben, Scotti, & Rabalais, 2003). He should also make certain that he is vetting these decisions with a supervisor or colleague.

The Likely Answer

If Jaco decides to look at his diagnosis again, he needs vetted instruments and a supervisor who will give him honest feedback. If he decides to go ahead with the diagnosis, he needs to help Victor find a reasonable option for treatment moving forward.

USE OF APPROPRIATE INSTRUMENTS: PART 1 (*YOU BETTER HAVE A* VALID *REASON FOR DOING THAT*)

Kurt is a clinical supervisor at a mental health clinic. Presenting concerns for clients at the clinic vary widely, though depression has been a common diagnosis as of late.

At supervision this week, two of Kurt's supervisees, Dave and Krist, report that they have developed a smartphone app to be used by clients at the clinic. The app measures depression, with five Likert scale items asking clients to rate their current mood using a continuum of "smiley and frowny faces." Per Dave and Krist, consumers will be prompted at random intervals throughout the day to rate their current mood, with a graph available at the end of each week that shows variations of their mood over time.

In describing the app further, Dave and Krist state that their intentions are to develop it more thoroughly here at the clinic, with the eventual hope of "going global" and offering an instrument that has normative data to contextualize scores.

They are requesting permission from Kurt to distribute the app to clients at the clinic, with the hope that it will (a) help the clients in understanding the ebb and flow of their own moods and utilize this information in session with their counselors and (b) develop a normative data set for the app's large scale roll out.

Questions for Discussion

1. *Is it acceptable to use an instrument that has not been vetted in a clinical mental health setting? Is there specific protocol that Kurt needs to follow?*
2. *Can employees of a mental health clinic engage in scale development and related research without an institutional review board (IRB)?*
3. *If Kurt did allow his employees to develop an instrument such as this, what considerations would need to be taken?*

Straight From the Code

1. **E.6.a. Appropriateness of Instruments.** Counselors carefully consider the validity, reliability, psychometric limitations, and appropriateness of instruments when selecting assessments and, when possible, use multiple forms of assessment, data, and/or instruments in forming conclusions, diagnoses, or recommendations.

Applying a Decision-Making Model: Garcia, Cartwright, Winston, and Borzuchowska's Transcultural Integrative Model

1. **Interpreting the situation through awareness and fact finding.** While the demographics of the clients served by the clinic are not directly indicated, community mental health clinics typically offer low-cost services to the general public. As such, developing a program of research with this population needs to be considered carefully, as the risk of exploitation is potentially high (i.e., clients may have few other options for treatment and need to feel as though they have agency in their own care). If Kurt chooses to allow his supervisees to develop this app, he will have to develop consent forms that describe—in language that all clients can clearly understand—the risks and benefits of participating in a project such as this.

   Additionally, Kurt must consider the degree to which a project such as this can be allowed to operate without oversight from an IRB. A staple within universities and colleges that conduct human subjects research, an IRB provides oversight of research to ensure the public's safety. While the risks of this particular project are likely very low, it should not be permitted to continue without an objective review of methodology and design.

2. **Formulating an ethical decision.** The code does not explicitly forbid development of measures by practicing clinicians, but it does state that psychometric properties of any instrument should be considered. This means that Kurt has the option to support or deny this project, though not without considering the pros and cons very carefully.

3. **Weighing competing, nonmoral values and affirming the course of action.** If Kurt allows the project to go on, the risk to clients at the clinic is—as previously stated—low, but not negligible. First, he would have to consider options for an independent review of the methodology (not required, but certainly recommended), as well as ensure support from the appropriate authorities at the clinic (e.g., chief executive officer, board members). Next, he would need to work with Dave and Krist to develop an informed consent protocol for the project that clearly outlines the benefits and risks of using this app, the intended purpose of the project, and allows for refusal to participate without

repercussions. Finally, he would have to be sure that both Dave and Krist are operating within their scope of competence, as he should not permit them to conduct a project such as this without adequate training. The information presented does not specify that Dave and Krist have advanced training in either research, statistics, or survey development.

Kurt should also take care to consider if clients are in any way being exploited as a function of the project. For disenfranchised populations in particular, the ability to decline consent can be complex. For example, some clients may not understand the specific details of the project, as a sample of the general population is unlikely to have a background in statistics such that they are aware of the nuances of validity and reliability. If the population served by the clinic includes individuals for whom English is not their first language, there would need to be assurances that the benefits and risks of the project are clearly explained in language that is understood by the clients. Kurt's ultimate concern should be the welfare of his clients, and—if he believes that there is a risk for exploitation of any kind, be it intentional or unintentional—he likely has an obligation to stop the project before it begins.

4. **Planning and executing the selected course of action.** If Kurt can determine that the project in no way compromises the mission of the clinic, does not exploit its clients, and has support from the higher ups at the clinic, he may be in the right to allow this project to continue. However, he would need to determine a way to verify that the methodology and design are acceptable. One possible option might be for Kurt to work with Dave and Krist to find a university in the area that would be interested in supporting the project. Junior professors (and academics in general) are always in need of publications, and the project might be better served by having more seasoned veterans provide support and assistance.

The Likely Answer

If Dave and Krist have the training and competence to pull this project off, the clinic's administrators support it, and he sees value beyond the general benefits to his staff, Kurt could potentially support the project. However, the case for doing so would be much stronger if a university or college with an IRB is involved.

USE OF APPROPRIATE INSTRUMENTS: PART 2 (*LOST IN TRANSLATION*)

Kurt was able to help Dave and Krist develop their app by linking them up with Professor Lovecraft at Misktonic University to provide oversight for the project. In addition to a successful rollout of the app (the Lovecraft Depression Scale and App), they were able to publish two papers in well-established counseling journals. The scale/app has been determined to be both reliable and valid in its current format.

The app has become a regular feature at the clinic, and Krist is now asking Kurt if he can make use of a Spanish version of the Lovecraft Depression Scale. This is to meet the needs of the growing Spanish-speaking population at the clinic.

Questions for Discussion

1. *Is developing a version of an established scale in another language acceptable?*
2. *What are the specific concerns relative to scale development that would have an impact on client welfare?*
3. *If Kurt did allow his employees to develop an instrument such as this, what considerations would need to be taken?*

Straight From the Code

1. **E.2.b. Appropriate Use.** Counselors are responsible for the appropriate application, scoring, interpretation, and use of assessment instruments relevant to the needs of the client, whether they score and interpret such assessments themselves or use technology or other services.

2. **E.6.a. Appropriateness of Instruments.** Counselors carefully consider the validity, reliability, psychometric limitations, and appropriateness of instruments when selecting assessments and, when possible, use multiple forms of assessment, data, and/or instruments in forming conclusions, diagnoses, or recommendations.

Applying a Decision-Making Model: Garcia, Cartwright, Winston, and Borzuchowska's Transcultural Integrative Model

1. **Interpreting the situation through awareness and fact finding.** In this case, we now know that the demographics of the clinic are in flux. Specifically, there has been an increase in the number of Spanish-speaking clients served by the clinic, and a rationale exists for refining existing assessment tools.

   However, there are specific protocols to be followed when developing an instrument in another language (Heppner, Wampold, Owen, Wang, & Thompson, 2015). In this case, it would be inappropriate to simply translate the questions from the English version to Spanish. Instead, a new version of the app would have to be first developed and then assessed with regard to reliability and validity.

2. **Formulating an ethical decision.** As in part 1 of this example, the code does not explicitly forbid development of measures by practicing clinicians, but it does state that psychometric properties of any instrument should be considered. This means that Kurt has the option to support or deny this project, though, again, not without considering the pros and cons very carefully.

3. **Weighing competing, nonmoral values and affirming the course of action.** Precedent has been set, such that a research project of this nature with university support may be allowed. Assuming that Dr. Lovecraft is willing to provide continued support for the project, the risk to clients at the clinic is low. In this case, there is established evidence based upon their history of scholarship that Dave and Krist are competent to manage a project of this magnitude.

   Still, Kurt should again consider if clients are in any way being exploited as a function of the project. The description of the case indicates that the demographics of the clinic have changed but that there has been no adjustment to the clinic's overall mission. Just because a research project *can* be implemented, that does not mean that it *should*, and concerns about clients' ability to consent to the project remain. If Kurt has any concerns that the clinic's clients are being exploited for the purposes of research, he should not support the project.

4. **Planning and executing the selected course of action.** As with part 1, if Kurt can determine that the project in no way compromises the mission of the clinic, does not exploit its clients, and has continued support from Dr. Lovecraft and the higher ups at the clinic, he may be in the right to allow this project to continue. It may also be acceptable if he decides that Dave and Krist are getting overzealous in their efforts to develop research projects and smartphone apps instead of helping clients.

The Likely Answer

If Dave and Krist have a solid plan, the clinic's administrators and Dr. Lovecraft support it, and he sees value beyond the general benefits to his staff, Kurt could potentially support a follow-up project.

UNSUPERVISED ASSESSMENT (*I PROBABLY SHOULD HAVE THOUGHT THIS THROUGH MORE CAREFULLY*)

Rochelle is a doctoral counseling student who is conducting research on resilience for her dissertation. She has decided to use the Resilience Scale (Wagnild, 2009) and has obtained the license with permission to use this assessment for her research for 1 year in both English and Spanish. In the license agreement, it states that Rochelle is the "licensee" and is the only one permitted to administer the assessment. She is planning to use this assessment with 300 12th-grade students in a local high school, about half of whom report greater comfort speaking Spanish than English. Rochelle has mapped out a schedule, so she will be able to get all the assessments done before the school year is over and her license to administer the instrument expires.

Rochelle, however, may have made a serious mistake in her planning: She does not speak Spanish. In her first run at administering these instruments to Spanish-speaking students, she struggles to explain the instrument effectively to the students.

There are 2 months left on the license to administer the scale and due to unforeseen issues with scheduling, Rochelle still has 66 students left to complete the assessment and most of them are Spanish speaking. As Rochelle does not speak Spanish, she is considering asking one of her bilingual peers in the counseling cohort if they would be willing to give the assessment to the remaining Spanish-speaking students on her behalf.

Questions for Discussion

1. *Since Rochelle is the licensee of the instrument, is she permitted to have someone else give the assessment, particularly if she is worried about her Spanish proficiency?*
2. *If Rochelle is in the room for the first few minutes does that count as administering the assessment?*
3. *Since Rochelle cannot speak Spanish, was it an appropriate idea for her to give the assessment in the first place?*

Straight From the Code

1. **E.7.a. Administration Conditions.** Counselors administer assessments under the same conditions that were established in their standardization. When assessments are not administered under standard conditions, as may be necessary to accommodate clients with disabilities, or when unusual behavior or irregularities occur during the administration, those conditions are noted in interpretation, and the results may be designated as invalid or of questionable validity.

2. **E.7.d. Unsupervised Assessments.** Unless the assessment instrument is designed, intended, and validated for self-administration and/or scoring, counselors do not permit unsupervised use.

Applying a Decision-Making Model: Garcia, Cartwright, Winston, and Borzuchowska's Transcultural Integrative Model

1. **Interpreting the situation through awareness and fact finding.** Rochelle is the only licensed person to administer the Resilience Scale. She has recognized her Spanish-speaking skills are not up to

par to give an assessment in this language, but she is in a time crunch to get all the assessments done. She likely realizes waiting until the last 2 months to address this was not a good decision, but she cannot go backward; she now has to decide what to do and how to get the assessments complete (or if she should continue them at all).

Despite her monolingualism, it is unlikely that Rochelle took this project on with the intention of negating these students. Having a peer who is bilingual is certainly an asset in this situation, particularly as she now realizes the extent to which her language skills are failing the project.

2. **Formulating an ethical decision.** The license on the instrument seems very straightforward: Rochelle is the licensee, which means that individuals not covered by the instrument are not permitted to act as administrators. If she passes this off to a peer, she leaves herself susceptible to legal action as she is breaking a contract, but she also may be violating the ACA Code's stipulations regarding the standardization of administration conditions.

   Though passing the assessments off to a peer that is not covered by the assessment license is likely not the best answer, Rochelle also needs to consider the implications of not including the Spanish-speaking students in her project. If she does not include these students, she may be negating the needs and experiences of an underserved population. She may need to consider what exceptions can be made to ensure that the project not only maintains acceptable standards of inquiry but also allows her to hear a range of experiences that represent the population of interest. Since Rochelle has been given access to both English and Spanish assessments, she might consider contacting the licensed owner of the Resilience Scale and ask what to do in relation to the Spanish-speaking students and/or seek licensing for her peer to conduct the assessments.

3. **Weighing competing, nonmoral values and affirming the course of action.** Rochelle has three basic options. First, she could attempt to administer the assessments on her own despite her limitations and simply note this as a limitation in her results. However, this could seriously compromise the study's findings in a way that might render the findings irrelevant. Second, she could ask her peer with more sufficient language skills to administer the instrument under her supervision. This would allow for a broader swath of data that likely represents the population of interest more effectively, but it would also violate the licensing agreement. Finally, she can contact the license's administrators to see if she can afford another license for her peer or if there is protocol established for administering the license under the supervision of another licensee. In this case, she may have definitive concern from the assessment's progenitors that the methodology of her study is significantly flawed.

4. **Planning and executing the selected course of action.** Though it may not provide her the answer she needs, Rochelle should likely start the process by reaching out to the administrators of the instrument to determine what (if any) options are available. If they suggest that supervised administration is appropriate, she still has to acknowledge this in her final write-up.

The Likely Answer

Rochelle should consult with the owner of the Resilience Scale and seek consultation as to how to handle this situation. If they allow her to conduct a supervised administration, she may be able to complete the study using this approach, though she should also state in her dissertation any limitations she experienced during the process of data collection. If this is not an option available, she may have to consider revamping the project completely.

REFRAINING FROM DIAGNOSIS (*WHAT'S IN A NAME?*)

Carmen is a counselor in private practice. She has been seeing Lucas as a client for the past year after he initially presented with depression and anxiety following a difficult breakup. Counseling has been going well overall in that Lucas indicates a strong connection with Carmen.

However, practical progress in the way of specific behavioral changes has been in short supply. Lucas continues to struggle with instability in his interpersonal relationships, with many of these problems being influenced by his feelings of self-importance, lack of empathy, and excessive need for admiration. Given both his current presentation and the fact that these problems seem to be a longstanding pattern, Carmen believes that Lucas may meet the criteria for narcissistic personality disorder (NPD).

As Lucas uses health insurance to pay for services, Carmen is required to indicate a diagnosis that will be submitted to his insurance company. Up to this point, she has used the more general category of "adjustment disorder with mixed anxiety and depression," but the insurance company has now indicated that they will no longer fund weekly counseling sessions for such a nebulous diagnosis.

Though NPD is the more appropriate diagnosis (and would likely provide additional funds for treatment), Carmen knows that Lucas will have access to whatever diagnosis she assigns. She is quite certain that her labeling him as narcissistic will not bode well for treatment.

Questions for Discussion

1. *Should Carmen just be honest with Lucas and assign him the appropriate diagnosis? Should she tell Lucas this information in advance?*

2. *Would it be better to assign Lucas a mood disorder instead (even if he does not technically meet the criteria)?*
3. *Is there a way to work with the insurance company to prevent Lucas from knowing his diagnosis?*

Straight From the Code

1. **E.5.d. Refraining From Diagnosis.** Counselors may refrain from making and/or reporting a diagnosis if they believe that it would cause harm to the client or others. Counselors carefully consider both the positive and negative implications of a diagnosis.

Applying a Decision-Making Model: Garcia, Cartwright, Winston, and Borzuchowska's Transcultural Integrative Model

1. **Interpreting the situation through awareness and fact finding.** This situation presents a unique challenge. First, Carmen needs to be certain that her diagnosis is correct. Mental health practitioners have a long history of gender bias in assigning diagnoses, particularly where personality disorders are concerned (e.g., Becker & Lamb, 1994), and NPD is far more commonly diagnosed in men than in women (Caligor, Levy, & Yeomans, 2015). The accuracy of the diagnosis also has a substantial impact on treatment: Some research has suggested that NPD-diagnosed individuals can present as a significant suicide risk given the likelihood of shame and related mood disorders (Ansell et al., 2015), though this has been contradicted by other inquiries (Coleman et al., 2017).

   Second, Carmen has to seriously consider the risk inherent in labeling Lucas as meeting the criteria for NPD. Personality disorders may carry stigma, and it is unlikely that Lucas will feel a greater sense of connection with Carmen if he finds she has labeled him as such.

2. **Formulating an ethical decision.** One option would be to simply submit the NPD diagnosis to the insurance company and hope that Lucas will not go through the trouble of looking this up. Another option would be to discuss this diagnosis with Lucas and inform him that this is what will be submitted to the insurance company for reimbursement (and it is what Carmen believes to be an accurate diagnosis). Another option would be to reach out to the insurance company directly to let them know of the concerns related to Lucas's access to his diagnosis.

3. **Weighing competing, nonmoral values and affirming the course of action.** Erroneously labeling Lucas as another diagnosis is obviously not an option, though she may want to carefully consider if

depression is a concern in this case given the rates of comorbidity. Submitting the diagnosis to the insurance company or simply sharing this outright with Lucas is potentially problematic as well. Assuming Carmen's diagnosis is accurate, it is highly unlikely that Lucas will agree with her. Reaching out to the insurance company to inform them of her concerns is likely the least harmful option.

4. **Planning and executing the selected course of action.** The insurance company may not be able to provide her an option to keep the diagnosis from the client, but—per the Code of Ethics—Carmen is within her right to refrain from providing a diagnosis that she worries may harm her client. In this case, instead of assigning the diagnosis of NPD (F60.81), Carmen might choose *Personality Disorder Not Otherwise Specified* (F60.9). This would technically be true as Lucas would meet the criteria for either, though it would be in her best interest to contact the insurance company directly and document their response.

The Likely Answer

Carmen should contact Lucas's insurance company, ask if it would be acceptable for billing purposes to use a more generic code, and document this contact in Lucas's chart.

IN-CLASS DISCUSSION AND EXERCISES

Group Discussion: Keeping Empathy Firmly in Place

In research, one of the more important ideas to keep firmly in place is empathy for the research participants. In conducting any study that involves human subjects, it is critical to ask yourself: If I were a participant in this research project, what would be my concerns? How comfortable would I feel with the procedures utilized for this project?

Take a moment and look at the articles published in the latest edition of a counseling journal (e.g., *Journal of Counseling and Development*, *Journal of Counseling Psychology*), and identify those that involve human subjects research. Read through the methods section, and try to imagine: If you were a participant, how would you feel about the line of inquiry or intervention being used here? What specific concerns might you have related to confidentiality, being compensated for your time, the invasiveness of the inquiry, or any aspect of the study's procedures?

Group Discussion: The Role of Deception

One consideration in some mental health research is the use of deception. For certain lines of inquiry, participants cannot be told about the entire nature of a specific project until it has concluded. For example, participants in a study exploring the efficacy of a particular counseling intervention will not be made aware of their enrollment in the treatment as usual (TAU) or experimental condition until the study's conclusion.

How should counseling researchers balance the need for disclosure versus the need for adherence to research protocol? Using the preceding example of a counseling intervention with either a wait list or TAU condition, how should researchers succinctly explain these concerns to their subjects? How comfortable would you feel if you later found that aspects of the research were not disclosed to you until the project's conclusion?

Role Play: Supervisors Need Supervision

Using the scenario described in *Supervisors Need Supervision*, role-play possible outcomes. Have one member play the role of KatieJane and another play the role of Crispin discussing the situation at hand. If you were KatieJane, how might you begin a dialogue? As Crispin, how might you actually feel or respond in the moment if KatieJane were to make efforts at resolving this matter directly?

Documentation: Problem, Data, Assessment, and Plan

Using the Problem, Data, Assessment, and Plan (PDAP) format, pick one of the cases and write a progress note indicating the following:
Problem: What were the presenting concerns of this particular interaction?
Data: What, objectively, has happened? Remember to write this without subjective language or interpretation.
Assessment: As the counselor or supervisor in question, what *should* be done? Be sure to demonstrate comprehensive use of the decision-making model in this section.
Plan: What *will* be done? Be sure to outline a comprehensive plan that relates to the decision-making model.

References

American Psychological Association. (2010). *Ethical principles of psychologists and code of conduct*. Washington, DC: Author.

Ansell, E. B., Wright, A. G., Markowitz, J. C., Sanislow, C. A., Hopwood, C. J., Zanarini, M. C., ... Grilo, C. M. (2015). Personality disorder risk factors for suicide attempts over 10 years of follow-up. *Personality Disorders: Theory, Research, and Treatment, 6*(2), 161. doi:10.1037/per0000089

Becker, D., & Lamb, S. (1994). Sex bias in the diagnosis of borderline personality disorder and posttraumatic stress disorder. *Professional Psychology: Research and Practice, 25*(1), 55. doi:10.1037/0735-7028.25.1.55

Bonino, J. L., & Hanna, F. J. (2018). Who owns psychopathology? The *DSM*: Its flaws, its future, and the professional counselor. *The Journal of Humanistic Counseling, 57*(2), 118–137. doi:10.1002/johc.12071

Caligor, E., Levy, K. N., & Yeomans, F. E. (2015). Narcissistic personality disorder: Diagnostic and clinical challenges. *American Journal of Psychiatry, 172*(5), 415–422. doi:10.1176/appi.ajp.2014.14060723

Coleman, D., Lawrence, R., Parekh, A., Galfalvy, H., Blasco-Fontecilla, H., Brent, D. A., ... Oquendo, M. A. (2017). Narcissistic personality disorder and suicidal behavior in mood disorders. *Journal of Psychiatric Research, 85*, 24–28. doi:10.1016/j.jpsychires.2016.10.020

Garcia, J. G., Cartwright, B., Winston, S. M., & Borzuchowska, B. (2003). A transcultural integrative model for ethical decision-making in counseling. *Journal of Counseling and Development, 81*(3), 268–277. doi:10.1002/j.1556-6678.2003.tb00253.x

Heppner, P. P., Wampold, B. E., Owen, J., Wang, K. T., & Thompson, M. N. (2015). *Research design in counseling* (4th ed.). Boston, MA: Cengage.

Hutchens, N., Block, J., & Young, M. (2013). Counselor educators' gatekeeping responsibilities and students' First Amendment rights. *Counselor Education and Supervision, 52*(2), 82–95. doi:10.1002/j.1556-6978.2013.00030.x

Kaplan, D. M., Francis, P. C., Hermann, M. A., Baca, J. V., Goodnough, G. E., Hodges, S., ... Wade, M. E. (2017). New concepts in the 2014 ACA code of ethics. *Journal of Counseling and Development, 95*(1), 110–120. doi:10.1002/jcad.12122

Kincheloe, J. L., Steinberg, S. R., & Gresson III, A. D. (1997). *Measured lies: The bell curve examined*. New York, NY: St. Martin's Press.

Ruggiero, K. J., Del Ben, K., Scotti, J. R., & Rabalais, A. E. (2003). Psychometric properties of the PTSD Checklist—Civilian version. *Journal of Traumatic Stress, 16*(5), 495–502. doi:10.1023/A:1025714729117

Wagnild, G. (2009). A review of the resilience scale. *Journal of Nursing Measurement, 17*(2), 105–113. doi:10.1891/1061-3749.17.2.105

Weiss, L. G., Saklofske, D. H., Coalson, D., & Raiford, S. E. (Eds.). (2010). *WAIS-IV clinical use and interpretation: Scientist-practitioner perspectives*. San Diego, CA: Academic Press.

Woodward, H. E., Taft, C. T., Gordon, R. A., & Meis, L. A. (2009). Clinician bias in the diagnosis of posttraumatic stress disorder and borderline personality disorder. *Psychological Trauma: Theory, Research, Practice, and Policy, 1*(4), 282. doi:10.1037/a0017944

CHAPTER 6

SUPERVISION, TEACHING, AND TRAINING
(SECTION F OF THE ACA CODE OF ETHICS)

INTRODUCTION

Cases in this section pertain to both counselor education and supervision throughout practice. At its core, counseling requires adherence to the basics of the scientist practitioner model both during training and after. This section highlights the ways in which colleges, universities, and supervisors can struggle at times in their efforts to meet the needs of students, faculty, and the public.

All cases will be assessed using Hill, Glaser, and Harden's (1998) feminist model for ethical decision-making.

HILL, GLASER, AND HARDEN'S FEMINIST MODEL

The feminist model for ethical decision-making is a theory-based model by Hill, Glaser, and Harden (1998). It represents an advanced method of considering identity, culture, and their combined impact on the decision-making process. Although linear in format, Hill et al. (1998) emphasize the fact that the outlined steps do not need to be implemented in any particular order to be effective, and consideration of consultation is a fundamental part of the process. For the process to work as intended, some steps may need to be revisited in certain circumstances. The model also encourages practitioners to consider not only the *rational evaluative* aspects of the process but also the clinician's instincts, the impact of the power differential in a therapeutic relationship, and the potential influence of counselor bias (Hill et al., 1998). The identities, opinions, and voices of both the client and the counselor are considered to be primary in the collaborative decision-making process between the two. The steps of the process are as follows:

1. **Recognizing a problem.** This is not yet defining parameters but first identifying that a dilemma exists.
2. **Defining the problem.** Define the specific parameters of the problem and the potential conflicts among the needs of the client, the needs of the profession, and the needs of the clinician(s).

3. **Developing solutions.** Develop a potential list of interventions that would theoretically resolve the dilemma.

4. **Choosing a solution.** Determine the best possible solution from the list developed, considering its fit and the degree to which it meets the needs of all parties involved.

5. **Reviewing the process.** Determine the procedures for defining what constitutes a successful resolution of the dilemma.

6. **Implementing and evaluating the decision.** Act on the solution that presents the least potential for harm and the best potential for resolution.

7. **Continuing reflection.** Once the decision has been enacted, continue to reflect on the outcomes, both upon retrospect and as a continued reflection of the decision's repercussions on the client(s), the profession, and the counselor(s).

INFORMED CONSENT AND CLIENT RIGHTS (*CAN YOU KEEP A SECRET?*)

DeeDee is a college counselor at a small university in a rural area. He is one of three counselors on staff, and his supervisor—Joey, the counseling center's director–sees him weekly for supervision. DeeDee enjoys his work with the college and feels a strong connection with Joey and the students he counsels.

In addition to supervision, Joey, DeeDee, and the rest of the counseling center staff attend a monthly meeting with the college's student life department. The meetings are typically a series of check-ins from each department, and Joey usually gives a brief report on behalf of the counseling center.

During today's meeting, Joey mentions an anecdote about one of DeeDee's clients. Specifically, during the check-in, he makes a joke about a client who had been struggling with personal hygiene: "We had a great month at the counseling center! No major problems with any of our clients, except for DeeDee—his regular Friday afternoon client keeps skipping showers and is stinking things up a bit. Other than that, it's been a great month!"

The joke gets a laugh from the group, but DeeDee feels uncomfortable with Joey making light of his client's struggles, particularly in a public forum.

Questions for Discussion

1. *Is it ever okay for clients to be discussed in detail during department meetings that contain employees not affiliated with the counseling center?*
2. *Is it acceptable to discuss clients in vague details such as this? Did Joey actually do anything wrong?*
3. *If DeeDee has concerns about Joey's behavior, what should he do?*

Straight From the Code

1. **F.1.c. Informed Consent and Client Rights.** Supervisors make supervisees aware of client rights, including the protection of client privacy and confidentiality in the counseling relationship. Supervisees provide clients with professional disclosure information and inform them of how the supervision process influences the limits of confidentiality. Supervisees make clients aware of who will have access to records of the counseling relationship and how these records will be stored, transmitted, or otherwise reviewed.

Applying a Decision-Making Model: Hill, Glaser, and Harden's Feminist Model

1. **Recognizing a problem.** Joey did not disclose any personal information about the client—no gender, no name, no specifics beyond the fact that a client DeeDee treats struggles with hygiene. However, it could certainly be argued that Joey behaved unprofessionally.
2. **Defining the problem.** The main problem here is likely Joey's lack of professionalism as well as the sense of betrayal DeeDee may feel in the aftermath of Joey's behavior. While confidentiality is not guaranteed in supervision the same way it is guaranteed in counseling, DeeDee likely assumed that the lion's share of the content revealed in these discussions would be kept in confidence.
3. **Developing solutions.** In this case, the options for DeeDee are to ignore what happened in the hopes that it was a one-time occurrence, discuss the matter directly with Joey, or reach out to Joey's direct supervisor.
4. **Choosing a solution.** If DeeDee ignores what happened, he runs the risk of not advocating for his clients and, by virtue of his omission, also runs the risk of setting a troubling precedent regarding the nature of client information discussed in supervision. If he discusses the matter directly with Joey, he runs the risk of compromising the relationship with his direct supervisor. The same is true if he discusses the matter with Joey's supervisor, as this will likely disrupt the relationship he has with Joey.
5. **Reviewing the process.** This is a challenging situation, but ultimately, DeeDee has to evaluate his own needs as a supervisee and the impact that Joey's behavior has on his clients. If he feels this oversight was enough that it warrants a discussion, he should probably start by addressing the matter with Joey directly.
6. **Implementing and evaluating the decision.** If DeeDee decides to go this route, he should carefully consider what would constitute *success*

in this case: An apology? An assurance that this will not happen again? A clarification of parameters in supervision? If the response he receives in this case is substandard (by his own definition), he could then escalate the situation to whomever oversees Joey.

7. **Continuing reflection.** DeeDee should be cautious in his approach, as he would not want to present the concern in an adversarial fashion if he chooses to confront Joey. However, he would also not want the matter to cause unaddressed resentment toward his supervisor. Whichever choice he makes, he needs to take caution in his approach and carefully monitor his relationship with Joey moving forward.

The Likely Answer

If he feels strongly enough about what happened, DeeDee should express his concerns to Joey. If he feels Joey's response is not enough, he could then reach out to Joey's supervisor.

IMPAIRMENT (THE PROCESS OF WEEDING OUT)

Al is a graduate student in a master's level counselor training program. His cohort is currently in the process of completing their practicum—the first direct experience with counseling for the majority of students. He has a close relationship with many of his fellow students but has lately developed a kinship with Matt, a member of his cohort who shares a lot of common interests in music and pop culture.

Prior to this week's group supervision, Matt and Al are outside smoking cigarettes and chatting about school. During the discussion, Al confides to Matt that these initial experiences with counseling make him nervous, particularly as the specifics of their program require them to videotape all of their sessions. Matt says that he feels the same way but that he usually "smokes a bowl before each session to calm down."

Questions for Discussion

1. *Does smoking marijuana before sessions fall under the umbrella of impairment?*
2. *Is Al obligated to report what Matt said to his supervisor?*
3. *What should Al say to Matt in response to this comment?*

Straight From the Code

1. **F.5.b. Impairment.** Students and supervisees monitor themselves for signs of impairment from their own physical, mental, or emotional problems and refrain from offering or providing professional services when such impairment is likely to harm a client or others. They notify

their faculty and/or supervisors and seek assistance for problems that reach the level of professional impairment, and, if necessary, they limit, suspend, or terminate their professional responsibilities until it is determined that they may safely resume their work.

Applying a Decision-Making Model: Hill, Glaser, and Harden's Feminist Model

1. **Recognizing a problem.** Unless Matt lives in a state where medical marijuana may be prescribed for anxiety, it is highly unlikely that he could provide justification for using marijuana before counseling sessions. Even if it were a state where marijuana was permitted for medicinal purposes, the clinic where he practices may have regulations in place regarding the use of medications during working hours. Whether this constitutes impairment would certainly be easier to determine if Matt had admitted to drinking alcohol before sessions, but it is unlikely that there will be sufficient justification for this behavior.

2. **Defining the problem.** Assuming Matt's behavior constitutes impairment, Al is now aware of this impairment and is obligated to respond in some fashion.

3. **Developing solutions.** Al has three options. He could simply acknowledge what Matt said and suggest that he not do this anymore. He could acknowledge what Matt said, ask that he not do this anymore, and ask that he provide some proof that he is attending counseling to address anxiety and his drug use. Or he could simply tell his supervisor what Matt said, either with Matt's knowledge or not.

4. **Choosing a solution.** Though the Code does indicate that resolutions of ethical dilemmas should be managed independently before escalating to the next level, it is unlikely that a resolution could be achieved in this case that would prove sufficient. If Al were to simply ask Matt to stop smoking marijuana before sessions, he would not be afforded any additional assurances that Matt had received help. If he asked Matt to provide proof of receiving help, this would likely go beyond the scope of his ability as a graduate student.

   If, however, he reaches out to his supervisor in the program, he runs the risk of hurting his relationship with Matt, in addition to reducing the likelihood that Matt will be honest with others during times of struggle in his work as a counselor. How to navigate this without harming Matt is complicated to say the least. Al would have to decide whether Matt would respond best with complete honesty and tell him immediately that he needs to discuss this with a supervisor or whether he would want to meet with a supervisor first to determine a course of action.

5. **Reviewing the process.** The option that best suits the situation is likely reaching out to a supervisor or faculty member at the university. In doing so, however, Al runs the risk of compromising his relationship with someone who is not just a peer, but a trusted friend. Al does indeed have agency in this situation, in that while he is technically obligated to respond in some fashion, he could certainly abide by his own morals and choose only to admonish Matt's behavior to Matt directly. It should also be noted that this would put him in a difficult situation if Matt's behavior were found out by another student or supervisor, particularly if it were determined that Al knew and did not intervene.

6. **Implementing and evaluating the decision.** As in the previous example, Al would first want to determine what *success* would be in trying to intervene at the most basic level first (i.e., admonishing his behavior and requesting that he get the necessary support). In this case, there does not seem to be a potential solution that Al could implement that would not either require him to act outside of his competence (e.g., directing him to substance abuse treatment) or put him in a position where he is forced to take the word of a friend that clients would not be harmed by his continuing behavior.

7. **Continuing reflection.** Cases such as this are particularly challenging. On one hand, the profession of counseling cannot advocate for a counselor to continue treating clients if they are impaired in some way. On the other, the profession should embrace its humanistic values such that impaired counselors receive support as opposed to being simply punished.

The Likely Answer

Al is faced with a difficult choice, as his actions affect both clients and his close friend. However, there seems to be limited options beyond mentioning Matt's comment to a supervisor or professor at the university.

SUPERVISORY RELATIONSHIP (*CAN WE JUST BE FRIENDS?*)

Francesca is a recent graduate of a counselor education program. She has just completed her postgraduate hours for her state license at a local drug and alcohol clinic where she worked as a counselor under the supervision of Marvin. Marvin is a licensed counselor who is 5 years senior to Francesca, and the two have met for weekly supervision over the course of the past 2 years.

At the completion of their final supervisory session, Marvin surprised Francesca by stating that he had romantic feelings for her. Specifically, he said that he had "dreamed for 2 years" about finally being able to ask her out on a date. Francesca, however, did not reciprocate his feelings. Despite enjoying their work together in supervision, she did not feel the same way and made her best effort to politely decline: "I really appreciate this, Marvin, but I would much rather we just stay friends."

Francesca and Marvin have been coworkers now for 3 months since the incident occurred, though Marvin refuses to speak with her or make eye contact since she declined his advance. This has made work difficult for Francesca at times, as staff meetings have become increasingly awkward and uncomfortable.

Questions for Discussion

1. *Was it okay for Marvin to ask Francesca out on a date? Is it ever acceptable for a counselor to become romantically involved with a former supervisor?*
2. *Though Marvin's behavior—refusing eye contact and conversation—could be argued as immature, is it in any way unethical? Does he have the right to manage his heartbreak however he sees fit?*
3. *Should Francesca reach out to one of her supervisors about all of this?*

Straight From the Code

1. **F.3.b. Sexual Relationships.** Sexual or romantic interactions or relationships with current supervisees are prohibited. This prohibition applies to both in-person and electronic interactions or relationships.

2. **F.3.c. Sexual Harassment.** Counseling supervisors do not condone or subject supervisees to sexual harassment.

Applying a Decision-Making Model: Hill, Glaser, and Harden's Feminist Model

1. **Recognizing a problem.** The Code states that romantic relationships with current supervisors are prohibited, but it says nothing about *former* supervisors. As such, it may have been acceptable for Marvin to disclose his feelings for Francesca, though his pattern of behaviors after she declined has made for an uncomfortable work environment. While he is no longer making advances toward her, he is still treating her unkindly in the aftermath of her rebutting his feelings.

2. **Defining the problem.** The question becomes whether Marvin's behaviors are serious enough to be considered sexual harassment. Though his intentions are likely stemming from his own feelings of heartache or insecurity, this is having an impact on Francesca's ability to do her job. The potential impact on Francesca's career should be underscored: Behaviors such as Marvin's can have adverse effects upon the careers of others, as this may facilitate job change that would affect career attainment over time (McLaughlin, Uggen, & Blackstone, 2017).

3. **Developing solutions.** Francesca has three options: She could not respond any further if she feels uncomfortable addressing Marvin or her superiors; she could make further attempts to address the issue with Marvin directly; or she could simply report her concerns to Marvin's direct supervisor(s).

4. **Choosing a solution.** As Marvin is refusing to speak with her, the likely solution in this case is to reach out to either his direct supervisor or the clinic's human resources department (if applicable) to make them aware of her concerns.

   Though it would seem ill advised for Francesca not to respond in any way, this is certainly an option. If she has other concerns related to her career that she fears may be adversely affected by confronting Marvin or his superiors, she reserves the right to handle this situation how she sees fit. While the Code might suggest the importance of trying to resolve concerns informally (in this case, trying to talk to Marvin first), Francesca is *not* obligated to do this if she feels threatened in any way by Marvin.

5. **Reviewing the process.** What option Francesca chooses is entirely up to her, though it is likely that any effort to reprimand Marvin for his behavior may lead to further unrest at work before things improve. However, a decision to *not* address this behavior could cause it to continue in perpetuity.

6. **Implementing and evaluating the decision.** What direction Francesca takes would likely be affected by her own level of comfort as well as what constitutes a successful outcome. Would she prefer not to have to have direct contact with Marvin anymore? Would she want them to be able to reestablish a friendly working relationship? In either case, how would success be defined?

7. **Continuing reflection.** If she does opt to address the problem with Marvin's superiors, the clinic where Francesca and Marvin work may wish to consider implementing policies regarding workplace intimacy.

The Likely Answer

Francesca is free to decide how this situation should be handled and should consider what would constitute *success* with whatever direction she chooses to take.

GATEKEEPING AND REMEDIATION (*REGROUPING*)

Ladybird is the director of a Council for Accreditation of Counseling and Related Educational Programs (CACREP)–accredited counseling program. One of the students in her program, Tom, has requested to speak with her as he has concerns about the group counseling class he is currently taking.

During the meeting, Tom discloses that he is struggling with the group experience component of the course. Specifically, he reports to have serious concerns about one of the group members, Jason, who identifies as gay. Tom states that he is Christian with "strong traditional values" and that he is completely uncomfortable with Jason's "lifestyle choice." He is requesting that he be transferred to a different section of the course.

When Ladybird asks for further clarification of Tom's values, he states that he has no intention of working with homosexual clients in his eventual practice, unless he can "help them find a way to change their lifestyle."

Questions for Discussion

1. *As these are Tom's personal values, is he within his right to request a transfer to a different section of the class?*
2. *Can Tom work as a counselor if his personal values are in direct contrast to the values of the profession?*
3. *How should Ladybird respond to all of this?*

Straight From the Code

1. **F.6.b. Gatekeeping and Remediation.** Through initial and ongoing evaluation, supervisors are aware of supervisee limitations that might impede performance. Supervisors assist supervisees in securing remedial assistance when needed. They recommend dismissal from training programs, applied counseling settings, and state or voluntary professional credentialing processes when those supervisees are unable to demonstrate that they can provide competent professional services to a range of diverse clients. Supervisors seek consultation and document their decisions to dismiss or refer supervisees for assistance. They ensure that supervisees are aware of options available to them to address such decisions.

Applying a Decision-Making Model: Hill, Glaser, and Harden's Feminist Model

1. **Recognizing a problem.** The Code states that supervisors of counselors may recommend dismissal from the program in cases where clinicians are incapable of demonstrating competence. In this case, Tom is clearly demonstrating incompetence as he is reportedly unwilling to work with clients who identify as gay unless he can assist them in changing their sexual identity. Conversion therapy (i.e., counseling intended to alter an individual's sexual identity from gay to straight)

has been disavowed by the majority of mental health organizations, as there is strong support for its potential to harm clients (Drescher et al., 2016).

2. **Defining the problem.** Tom has directly stated that his personal values would lead him to engage in actions that may potentially harm clients. This is a particularly complex problem as it has been the focus of several lawsuits in the United States. In the case of *Ward v. Wilbanks*, a student sued a counselor education program after being dismissed for indicating the intention to refuse treatment of clients identifying as gay (Kaplan, 2014). A similar lawsuit occurred at Augusta State University, when a student was dismissed for refusing to take part in remedial procedures in the aftermath of stating outright refusal to treat clients identifying as homosexual (Herlihy, Herman, & Greden, 2014). Though both of these dismissals were upheld in court, Ladybird is presented with the concern that advocating for the values of her profession could potentially result in litigation.

3. **Developing solutions.** There seems to be only one option at present: Consult with the program staff at the university (e.g., Tom's advisor, the faculty steering committee) as well as the administrative staff who oversee the department and program (e.g., the academic dean). Assuming all are in agreement and university policy supports it, Tom may be provided the option to engage in remediation procedures to ensure that his values are in keeping with those of the profession. As in the Augusta State case, the program could offer him the opportunity to engage in LGBTQ-related readings, lectures, and other activities with reflection exercises to explore his biases and the impact they may have on his work. If Tom refuses this option, he may face dismissal from the program.

4. **Choosing a solution.** Ladybird might, depending on Tom's presentation, view the situation as an isolated incident, discuss her concerns with Tom directly, and then clarify with Tom if he is absolutely certain that his values prevent him from behaving ethically. It is important to remember that Tom is permitted to have his own values and beliefs, but only if he can ensure that they will not hurt the clients he sees.

5. **Reviewing the process.** It will be important for Ladybird to treat Tom with respect and compassion throughout this process. Discussions related to personal beliefs and values can be challenging, and it is in everyone's best interest to try and keep the discourse as civil as possible. This could also potentially decrease the likelihood of a lawsuit if concerns can be resolved amicably.

6. **Implementing and evaluating the decision.** One of the problems faced in a situation such as this is that what constitutes belief and value are, essentially, abstraction. Ladybird could implement a series of personal reflection exercises for Tom, and Tom could indicate in

writing that his values were in fact a fit with the profession of counseling. However, the outcomes of this could only be measured by observing Tom's eventual behaviors as a professional counselor.

7. **Continuing reflection.** It would be important for the program to work in conjunction with the university to ensure that all promotional material clearly states the program's mission and values as it relates to professional counseling. A long-term resolution would be to avoid matters such as this happening in the future by discouraging students from applying if the program (and the field) is not in keeping with its own values.

The Likely Answer

Ladybird should demonstrate compassion in her efforts to better understand the extent to which Tom's values are (or are not) in keeping with the profession and work with the department and university to develop a remediation plan if necessary. If Tom is not amenable to these plans, dismissal from the program may be appropriate.

USE OF CASE EXAMPLES (*THIS IS GETTING PRETTY META*)

Indigo is a graduate student in a counselor education program in a rural area. This semester, she is taking a course titled Counseling Theories and Interventions taught by Dr. Octavius. Dr. Octavius is known both for his work as a professor and for his private practice in town where he sees individuals, couples, and families for counseling. In fact, Indigo is somewhat excited to have him as a professor, as her close friend Aeon has been seeing him for individual counseling for several years now and insists that he is a "genius."

A major component of the course contains case examples, as Dr. Octavius regularly demonstrates the nuances of counseling theories using examples from clients he has treated. In today's lecture, however, Indigo is quite certain that the case example being discussed is actually Aeon. While he uses a pseudonym in the description, the overview includes very specific information about Aeon's dating and personal life such that it would *have* to be her. At one point, he even discusses some of his own feelings of countertransference toward this client, indicating that he often finds her "annoying."

Questions for Discussion

1. *Is it acceptable to include case examples from actual clinical practice for the purposes of education?*
2. *Did Dr. Octavius do a sufficient job in safeguarding his client's identity?*
3. *How should Indigo respond to all of this? Should she say anything to Aeon? Should she talk to Dr. Octavius?*

Straight From the Code

1. **F.7.f. Use of Case Examples.** The use of client, student, or supervisee information for the purposes of case examples in a lecture or classroom setting is permissible only when (a) the client, student, or supervisee has reviewed the material and agreed to its presentation or (b) the information has been sufficiently modified to obscure identity.

Applying a Decision-Making Model: Hill, Glaser, and Harden's Feminist Model

1. **Recognizing a problem.** The Code states that such examples are acceptable in cases where the client gave permission (it does not appear that Aeon did so) *or* in cases where the presenting information is modified such that identity is obscured. In this case, it seems the problem is that Dr. Octavius did not obscure the details enough such that the client—or in this case, someone who knows the client well—would be unaware of whom the case was describing. This is an important consideration, as skills-based classes such as these would likely benefit tremendously from real-world experiences described by the instructor. However, a good rule of thumb should be that if the client were to read the case example, the demographic information and specifics of the case must be altered such that the client would be unaware that this case was about them (unless they consent to the example being used for educational purposes).
2. **Defining the problem.** Indigo, a counselor-in-training, is aware that her professor has potentially violated a client's confidentiality by not obscuring information adequately. However, it is possible (albeit unlikely) that Aeon has given consent for this example to be used.
3. **Developing solutions.** One option would be for Indigo to discuss her concerns with Dr. Octavius. She could meet him after class, indicate that she knows Aeon is a client of his, and express concern about his adherence to confidentiality. A second option would be to discuss her concerns with Aeon directly by explaining that confidentiality appeared to have been violated during the course of a lecture. A third option would be to reach out to one of Dr. Octavius's supervisors to discuss her concerns.
4. **Choosing a solution.** If Indigo opts to talk to Dr. Octavius, she runs the risk of compromising her performance in the course. As stated in previous examples, informal resolution of ethical concerns is preferable but is often compromised by practical concerns (e.g., reprimanding someone who has evaluative authority). Frankly, this concern is evident in all of her available options, as Dr. Octavius will at some point be aware of a complaint at his expense made by a student, and the connection to Indigo would likely be difficult to miss.

However, Aeon deserves autonomy in this case, as she is likely the client who has been victimized. As such, Indigo might begin the process by confronting Aeon first and asking how she would like to proceed.

5. **Reviewing the process.** If Aeon claims that she has no interest in pursuing the matter, this is her prerogative, and Indigo will need to honor that. If, however, she has concerns about the content of this disclosure, she is well within her right to choose to confront Dr. Octavius on her own or to request Aeon's support in contacting his supervisors at the university.

6. **Implementing and evaluating the decision.** This situation is complicated for many reasons, but one in particular stands out: What is an acceptable resolution? If Aeon is aware that her confidence has been violated by her counselor, what will allow her to feel as though the matter has been resolved? What has been made public cannot be taken back at this point. Would an apology suffice? Would she need to see Dr. Octavius sanctioned for his actions? Is there anything he could say or do in response to these accusations that might make this right? Is this the end of counseling between Aeon and Dr. Octavius?

7. **Continuing reflection.** If the program is involved in this matter (assuming Aeon approves of the decision to reach out to the university directly), it would likely be recommended that the university review its faculty handbooks and related policies. Administrative faculty and related members may use this as an opportunity to remind faculty about the importance of adherence to basic ethical principles in their teaching and supervision.

The Likely Answer

Indigo should reach out to Aeon, let her know what she heard, and work with Aeon to determine the course of action that best meets her needs.

RELATIONSHIPS WITH FORMER STUDENTS (*CAN ANYBODY FIND ME SOMEBODY TO LOVE?*)

Carmela is a newly tenured faculty member at a small liberal arts college where she teaches in the counselor education program. While proud of her recent accomplishment, she is quick to admit that the 5 years she has spent at this institution have been lonely. In addition to being lost in her work, the college is at least 2 hours by car to any major metropolitan area, all of which has made dating a real challenge.

A glimmer of hope (mixed with confusion) presents itself when Carmela finally meets Kayita. Though Kayita is a student in the department, she felt an instant connection with her. The two met for coffee after class on one occasion, ostensibly to talk about research interests and Kayita's applications to doctoral programs. However, Carmela ended the meeting abruptly when she began to realize they had been chatting for 2 hours about their personal lives and had not once discussed anything related to school. As she saw that her feelings for Kayita were veering toward the romantic, she began to limit their contact outside of school-related concerns.

She could not stop from thinking about her, though. Throughout the 2 years Kayita remained as a student in the program, and a student in four of her classes, Carmela would have to admit that she has been daydreaming about Kayita constantly. To make matters more complicated, Kayita has regularly joked with her about how she "can't wait until we're finally colleagues so we can get coffee again."

Graduation is now approaching, and Carmela is considering asking her on an official date following the college's commencement ceremony.

Questions for Discussion

1. *Is it ever acceptable for an educator to date a former student?*
2. *Assuming Carmela decides to ask Kayita out on a date, should she reach out to someone in the college to make sure this is in keeping with the institution's policies?*
3. *What if Kayita says no?*

Straight From the Code

1. **F.10.a. Sexual or Romantic Relationships.** Counselor educators are prohibited from sexual or romantic interactions or relationships with students currently enrolled in a counseling or related program and over whom they have power and authority. This prohibition applies to both in-person and electronic interactions or relationships.

2. **F.10.c. Relationships with Former Students.** Counselor educators are aware of the power differential in the relationship between faculty and students. Faculty members discuss with former students' potential risks when they consider engaging in social, sexual, or other intimate relationships.

Applying a Decision-Making Model: Hill, Glaser, and Harden's Feminist Model

1. **Recognizing a problem.** It does not appear that Carmela has behaved unethically based upon the overview provided thus far. She is currently pining for a (soon to be) former student, though feelings in and of themselves are not an ethical violation. Regardless of what the

Code and the institution's policies state, she is considering the possibility of engaging in a romantic relationship with someone she once taught and assigned grades to.

2. **Defining the problem.** The Code indicates that romantic relationships with current students are prohibited. It does not, however, clarify at what point a student earns the designation "former"—Is it immediately after final grades are submitted? Immediately after graduation? What if Kayita decides to reenter the program to pursue additional training or certification of some kind?

3. **Developing solutions.** One option would be to simply ignore her feelings and refuse to engage in a romantic relationship with a student, former or otherwise. Another option would be to determine what constitutes the best possible course of action in her efforts to engage in a romantic relationship with a former student/recent graduate of her program.

4. **Choosing a solution.** Not pursuing this relationship may seem heartbreaking to Carmela, but it is a viable option. Though the Code of Ethics for counselors, as well as policy for most universities in the United States, do not forbid relationships with former students, the risks in doing so include difficulty navigating changes in the relationship dynamic; poor distinctions between pursuing and harassing; and the ongoing potential for litigation if the relationship sours (Flaherty, 2019).

   However, Kayita has recourse to pursue a romantic relationship if she chooses. The counterargument to the aforementioned concerns about relationships with former students has been simply put: Consenting adults (including faculty and former students) should have the right to engage in relationships with whomever they choose (McArthur, 2017).

5. **Reviewing the process.** If Carmela decides *not* to pursue a relationship with Kayita, the process ends here, though she might examine other avenues for pursuing romantic relationships despite her physical isolation. If she *does* decide to ask her out on a date, she has to first consider the point at which her role as instructor officially ends. If, for example, she turns in her final grades and then decides to ask her out on a date, what would happen if Kayita decides to protest the grade that has been issued? It may be warranted for Carmela to reach out to her department chair, dean, or possibly the college's human resources department to determine what policies exist regarding relationships with former students.

6. **Implementing and evaluating the decision.** As stated earlier, the evaluation of the decision moving forward is an important step. If Carmela does not decide to pursue a relationship, it would be important

for her to consider what aspects of this relationship with a student had caused her such temptation. She should also determine what other options exist for pursuing a relationship if she intends to stay in the area.

If Carmela does ask Kayita on a date and she says yes, how will they navigate the terrain of this new relationship moving forward? Carmela was once in a position where she held authority over Kayita, such that she was seen as a master and Kayita was seen as a novice; now the expectation (presumably) is that they will be entering a new relationship as equals. Is this possible? How will either adjust to a complete change in the dynamics of power in this new relationship?

Finally, how will Carmela manage this situation moving forward if Kayita rejects her advance? From the description of events, it seems unlikely that Carmela is misreading a mutual attraction from Kayita, but what if she is? What if Kayita offers a yes in response to this request but is only doing so out of a sense of obligation or a misunderstanding that this is an invite for networking from a colleague?

7. **Continuing reflection.** Whatever path she chooses (and whatever Kayita offers in response), Carmela has much to consider moving forward. If a relationship with Kayita does manifest itself, navigating a change in dynamics such as this will be complicated business to say the least. If not, she has much to consider about how to manage relationships moving forward if she intends to stay at a college in a small town.

The Likely Answer

If Carmela is intent on pursuing this relationship, she should first check with the college to determine the relevant constraints and procedures. If Kayita says yes, they both have a lot to think about moving forward regarding the changing dynamics of their relationship.

LIMITATIONS (*THE* UN-*NATURAL*)

Kaprea is a counselor educator at a large public university. As part of her regular teaching load, she is responsible once a semester for the basic skills course. She has been teaching this class for almost 6 years now, and it is one of her favorites. She genuinely enjoys watching students engage in the work of counseling for the first time.

However, Graham, a first-year student in the program, has proven to be something of a challenge. He is nervous and shy, often appearing very uncomfortable in the most basic of interactions with faculty and other students. Problems with his demeanor are persistent such that other professors have discussed his interpersonal skills (and their concerns) during recent faculty meetings.

It is his tapes of mock counseling vignettes that have Kaprea seriously worried, though—he is required to complete three for the course. In the first, he appeared to be having a moderate anxiety attack as he stumbled through the most basic of introductory questions and pleasantries; he did not even demonstrate any of the basic skills discussed in class. Kaprea assumed this was just nerves, gave him ample feedback, discussed her concerns with faculty during their regular program meeting, and offered Graham additional support. In response, Graham stated that he struggles with anxiety but denied her offer to seek support through the university's counseling center. In his second tape, however, his anxiety and interpersonal difficulties seemed even worse; the tape ended after 5 minutes of nervous dialogue.

Kaprea schedules a meeting to discuss her concerns with Graham. While he again admits to her that he has struggled with social anxiety for much of his life, he states that it has always been his dream to help others overcome similar challenges. He once more refuses her referral to university counseling services. In fact, he is surprisingly recalcitrant throughout the meeting, indicating that he is aware of his struggles but that it is the program's job to provide him with better training and additional support.

Graham has one more tape to complete for the class. Kaprea is genuinely concerned that, without counseling support to address his social anxiety, he will be unable to pass the course.

Questions for Discussion

1. *Is it ever acceptable to dismiss a student from a training program if he or she struggles to provide basic counseling services?*
2. *Is there additional support that Kaprea could offer beyond feedback and referrals for treatment to address his ongoing anxiety?*
3. *Does Graham's admission of a mental health condition have any impact on how this matter should be resolved?*

Straight From the Code

1. **F.9.b. Limitations.** Counselor educators, through ongoing evaluation, are aware of and address the inability of some students to achieve counseling competencies. Counselor educators do the following:

   1. assist students in securing remedial assistance when needed.

2. Seek professional consultation and document their decision to dismiss or refer students for assistance.

3. Ensure that students have recourse in a timely manner to address decisions requiring them to seek assistance or to dismiss them and provide students with due process according to institutional policies and procedures.

Applying a Decision-Making Model: Hill, Glaser, and Harden's Feminist Model

1. **Recognizing a problem.** In short, Graham's counseling skills are a problem. Regardless of what mental health conditions he struggles with, the fact remains that he is having a hard time meeting the program's basic criteria. Worse yet, he has refused referrals for help to remedy the situation.

2. **Defining the problem.** The Americans with Disabilities Act (ADA, 1990) makes it illegal for an employer to fire a person as a result of a medical condition, and social anxiety, assuming Graham has documented evidence to verify he meets the relevant criteria, likely qualifies as a medical condition. More importantly, it would definitely be in direct contrast to the wellness-based principles of the counseling profession to dismiss a student from training as a result of a mental health concern.

   However, Graham's refusal to accept support for this condition creates a unique problem. Thus far, Kaprea has provided assistance and consulted with her peers, both of which are in keeping with the American Counseling Association (ACA) Code of Ethics. She has not, however, allowed Graham the appropriate time to address these concerns, as he has only completed two of the three required assignments.

3. **Developing solutions.** Dismissing Graham from the program seems an unlikely option, due to both legal concerns and adherence to the wellness principles of the counseling profession. Kaprea could simply ignore the matter, confident in the fact that she has offered Graham support and feedback that he has refused (and, subsequently, issue a failing grade for the course). She could also wait until the third tape to see if Graham improves; if he does not, she could work with the department to offer an incomplete grade so that he can retake the course.

4. **Choosing a solution.** Requiring a student to attend counseling does create some amount of legal risk, but providing Graham the opportunity to complete his third tape is a sensible starting point.

5. **Reviewing the process.** Kaprea will have to provide Graham with clear and concise feedback to ensure that he has all the required information to successfully complete the assignment. It may be recommended that she work closely, and document all of her interactions, with the program directors or chair as well as the school's disability support services office to ensure that she is providing reasonable accommodations and support.

6. **Implementing and evaluating the decision.** It would also likely be helpful for Kaprea to have another meeting with Graham to ask what

he feels the program could provide in the way of additional assistance. It would be important for Graham both to feel as though the university faculty have heard his requests for additional assistance and to ensure that support has been provided.

7. **Continuing reflection.** When students struggle to make use of the education and support provided, it can be a very frustrating experience. Kaprea should likely take the time to process this with her supervisor and other faculty members as appropriate.

The Likely Answer

Kaprea should meet with Graham to ask what support he feels he requires, discuss the matter with her chair and/or program director as appropriate, and document all of these interactions. If Graham is unable to pass the class, it may be appropriate to offer him a chance to retake the course.

IN-CLASS DISCUSSION AND EXERCISES

Group Discussion: Recognizing Potential Tripping Points (Supervisors)

Think about your own work history and your potential *tripping points* related to interactions with supervisors. Who have been the supervisors you got along with? Who were the ones you struggled with? Have there been specific personalities who triggered you in some way? Were there specific work-related concerns that caused you to get upset more easily than others?

Group Discussion: Difficult Conversations (Supervisors)

A hallmark of the cases in this section is the idea that some conversations can be both challenging and uncomfortable. Confronting supervisors, directly or indirectly, is never enjoyable, and devising practical methods for doing so can get pretty abstract.

Imagine you had to confront your current supervisor for making an inappropriate comment about one of your clients during a staff meeting. How would you go about this? What would you do to prepare for this conversation? Is there anything practically that you could do in advance of this discussion? Are you the type who prepares a script in advance? Do you do better with improvisation? Are there supervisors whom you would have an easier time doing this with? Why?

Role Play: The Process of Weeding Out

Using the scenario described in *The Process of Weeding Out*, role-play possible outcomes. Have one member play the role of Al and another play the role of Matt discussing the situation at hand. If you were Al, how might you begin a dialogue? As Matt, how might you actually feel or respond in the moment if Al were to make efforts at resolving this matter directly?

Documentation: Problem, Data, Assessment, and Plan

Using the Problem, Data, Assessment, and Plan (PDAP) format, pick one of the cases and write a progress note indicating the following:
Problem: What were the presenting concerns of this particular interaction?
Data: What, objectively, has happened? Remember to write this without subjective language or interpretation.
Assessment: As the counselor or supervisor in question, what *should* be done? Be sure to demonstrate comprehensive use of the decision-making model in this section.
Plan: What *will* be done? Be sure to outline a comprehensive plan that relates to the decision-making model.

References

Americans with Disabilities Act of 1990, Pub. L. No. 101-336, 104 Stat. 328 (1990).

Drescher, J., Schwartz, A., Casoy, F., McIntosh, C. A., Hurley, B., Ashley, K., … Mattson, M. R. (2016). The growing regulation of conversion therapy. *Journal of Medical Regulation, 102*(2), 7–12. doi:10.30770/2572-1852-102.2.7

Flaherty, C. (2019). Former student, fair game? *Inside Higher Ed.* Retrieved from https://www.insidehighered.com/news/2019/05/22/institutions-generally-dont-have-provisions-against-professors-dating-students-they

Herlihy, B. J., Hermann, M. A., & Greden, L. R. (2014). Legal and ethical implications of using religious beliefs as the basis for refusing to counsel certain clients. *Journal of Counseling and Development, 92*(2), 148–153. doi:10.1002/j.1556-6676.2014.00142.x

Hill, M., Glaser, K., & Harden, J. (1998). A feminist model for ethical decision making. *Women & Therapy, 21*(3), 101–121. doi:10.1300/J015v21n03_10

Kaplan, D. M. (2014). Ethical implications of a critical legal case for the counseling profession: *Ward v. Wilbanks*. *Journal of Counseling and Development, 92*(2), 142–146. doi:10.1002/j.1556-6676.2014.00140.x

McArthur, N. (2017). Relationships between university professors and students: Should they be banned? *Ethics and Education, 12*(2), 129–140. doi:10.1080/17449642.2017.1293922

McLaughlin, H., Uggen, C., & Blackstone, A. (2017). The economic and career effects of sexual harassment on working women. *Gender & Society, 31*(3), 333–358. doi:10.1177/0891243217704631

CHAPTER 7

RESEARCH AND PUBLICATION (SECTION G OF THE ACA CODE OF ETHICS)

INTRODUCTION

Research is not required as part of counseling practice. However, many counselors work exclusively in academic settings, and all counselors are obligated to stay informed of research relevant to the profession as well as understand the basics of ethics pertaining to research. Cases in this section highlight the specific components of ethical counseling research and related complications.

All cases will be assessed using Jacob, Roth, Cilento, and Stoler's (2015) model for making an ethical decision.

JACOB, ROTH, CILENTO, AND STOLER'S MODEL (2015)

The ethical decision-making model proposed by Jacob, Roth, Cilento, and Stoler (2015) draws from the social constructivist model by Cottone and the transcultural model from Garcia, Cartwright, Winston, and Borzuchowska (2003) and also focuses on the utility of supervision and clinical acumen. Like many other models, this is a step-by-step process, though this approach emphasizes directness and simplicity:

1. **Recognize the ethical dilemma and be aware of bias hotspots.** Counselors should be aware of what dilemma has been presented and the extent to which their own bias(es) may be triggered. The authors emphasize the importance of working to be mindful of potential decision-making tripping points before they occur.

2. **Practice mindful awareness.** The ultimate goal is reducing bias and checking emotions throughout the decision-making process. Ethical decision-making requires care and thoughtfulness, and counselors need to ensure that they carefully consider their internal experiences as well as the external experience of the dilemma.

3. **Reference the Code of Ethics.** Counselors are expected to reference the Code during the decision-making process. This can occur at the time of the dilemma or in the aftermath to ensure they are adhering to the standards of the profession.

4. **Consider alternative options.** It is suggested that *devil's advocate* be a regular aspect of the decision-making process and that all potential options are

considered or explored. The authors highlight the importance of exploring options that challenge their initial assumptions and instincts as well as those that support them.

5. **Consult as needed.** The authors recommend consulting not just with peers or supervisors who will tell a counselor what they *want* to hear, but also with those who may tell them what they *need* to hear. As with step 4, the concern is ensuring that initial assumptions are challenged as well as explored.

DUPLICATE SUBMISSIONS (*SPRAY AND PRAY*)

Clement is a brand-new professor in his first semester at a highly regarded institution that values productivity as part of the process to tenure. For his dissertation, he completed one study: a qualitative exploration of ethical decision-making in newly licensed counselors. This year, his former adviser/dissertation chair has suggested he submit this same project to one academic journal, a short version of the results to two counseling-themed magazines, one state conference, one national conference, and one regional conference. Clement likes the idea of multiple submissions but is uncertain if it is acceptable to submit the same project to various outlets.

Questions for Discussion

1. *Is it okay to submit the same research to numerous outlets?*
2. *Should any of these outlets be made aware of the fact that he is submitting to other outlets?*
3. *Even if Clement is not violating any specific ethical codes, is this practice beneficial to the profession overall?*

Straight From the Code

1. **G.5.g. Duplicate Submissions.** Counselors submit manuscripts for consideration to only one journal at a time. Manuscripts that are published in whole or in substantial part in one journal or published work are not submitted for publication to another publisher without acknowledgment and permission from the original publisher.

Applying a Decision-Making Model: Jacob, Roth, Cilento, and Stoler's Model

1. **Recognize the ethical dilemma and be aware of bias hotspots.** In this case, Clement needs to be aware of his own need to publish, present, and stay afloat in the world of academia. The expression *publish*

or perish refers to the pressures of academics to consistently produce work that is novel, often at the expense of adherence to the rigors of science (Grimes, Bauch, & Ioannidis, 2018). Clement likely values his job and may be inclined to engage in the necessary mental gymnastics to justify his actions if they are in support of his efforts to stay employed as a professor.

2. **Practice mindful awareness.** As such, Clement needs to examine his decision-making very carefully. Is there evidence to suggest that he *needs* to publish at this rate in order to ensure tenure? Universities often outline the specific requirements for tenure in faculty handbooks, and it would be important for Clement to determine the extent to which his fears are justifiable. Is this drive to publish and present in numerous scholarly outlets driven by practical concerns, or is it in some way connected to Clement's (or his former adviser/chair's) insecurities?

3. **Reference the Code of Ethics.** The Code only suggests that it is unethical to submit to more than one academic journal at a time. In this case, Clement has made no efforts to go beyond this requirement: He is submitting to numerous scholarly outlets, but only one of them is identified as an academic journal.

4. **Consider alternative options.** The concern with this behavior, submitting the same project to numerous outlets, is that it conflates reputability of a project with the number of lines a professor has on their curriculum vita. Submitting the same project over and over again may fill the necessary requirements for tenure, but it does not necessarily suggest the work itself to be of significant value. Alternatively, it could be argued that dissemination of results is akin to marketing, in that it is the responsibility of the study's progenitors to find ways to make their work available to the public.

5. **Consult as needed.** In this case, Clement has consulted with his former adviser and dissertation chair. However, it might be better to check in with his current department chair to see if he or she has any ideas about what constitutes an acceptable series of publication for tenure. Divorced of the ethics of numerous submissions, this process of *double dipping* (i.e., presenting the same project in numerous forums) may be viewed with skepticism by the department or tenure and promotion committee.

The Likely Answer

Clement has not violated any specific ethical parameter as of yet, but he should probably check with his chair to be sure he is on the right track.

STUDENT RESEARCH AND AGREEMENT OF CONTRIBUTORS (*PARDON ME FOR A SECOND, BUT I'M JUST GOING TO TAKE YOUR CREDIT*)

Malachi is a doctoral student finishing his dissertation at Miskatonic University under his adviser Dr. Herbert West. His dissertation examines the utility of dream analysis in grief counseling, and Dr. West was instrumental in helping him collect the data. As Malachi is in the process of applying to tenure-track faculty positions, he is working with Dr. West to publish his findings in a top-tier counseling journal with Dr. West as a second author.

Malachi submitted a first draft of his findings to the *Journal of Dream Research*. The feedback is surprisingly critical, suggesting that his statistical analysis was inherently flawed. Distraught, he shows the feedback to Dr. West, who assures him he will "fix it," as he has a strong background in a specific statistical procedure that he believes will improve the article. Malachi is grateful for the help and gives Dr. West all of his raw data.

Six weeks later, Dr. West has completed a new draft of the paper and emails it to Malachi. Malachi reads the draft and is impressed overall with Dr. West's improvements. However, he is surprised to find that Dr. West has now listed himself as first author and Malachi as second author.

Questions for Discussion

1. *Was Dr. West justified in listing himself as the lead author?*
2. *Should Malachi tell Dr. West that he is concerned with this development? How could he discuss these concerns in a way that is tactful but thoroughly expresses his dissatisfaction with the outcome?*
3. *Even if Dr. West was justified in taking lead authorship, might there have been a better way to address this with Malachi?*

Straight From the Code

1. **G.5.e. Agreement of Contributors.** Counselors who conduct joint research with colleagues or students/supervisors establish agreements in advance regarding allocation of tasks, publication credit, and types of acknowledgment that will be received.

2. **G.5.f. Student Research.** Manuscripts or professional presentations in any medium that are substantially based on a student's course papers, projects, dissertations, or theses are used only with the student's permission and list the student as lead author.

Applying a Decision-Making Model: Jacob, Roth, Cilento, and Stoler's Model

1. **Recognize the ethical dilemma and be aware of bias hotspots.** Malachi is likely feeling somewhat hurt and/or betrayed by Dr. West, as his feelings about his research and his adviser are likely to be strong. However, it will be important for him to keep these strong feelings in check to the best of his abilities as he attempts to resolve the matter with Dr. West. It is important for the sake of general decorum to avoid getting angry with an academic mentor, but it is also a good rule of thumb to maintain relationships with potential references.

2. **Practice mindful awareness.** Malachi should probably take a day or so to examine his feelings before responding to Dr. West. If he is angry, is it more directed at Dr. West taking the credit or more directed at himself for not having the statistical savvy to make the necessary edits on the article? Can he find a way to manage his anger and related emotions such that they will not compromise his relationship with Dr. West?

3. **Reference the Code of Ethics.** The Code is clear that Malachi should likely have been afforded first authorship if he was the driving force behind the publication (G.5.f), though the extent to which the paper is based on Malachi's dissertation in the aftermath of Dr. West's edits is unclear. It may be that Dr. West's edits to the article were substantial to the point that the project is almost new. It seems clear that authorship and credit should have been established in advance (G.5.e.), though the paper has yet to be submitted for publication.

4. **Consider alternative options.** Malachi has two basic options: Either confront Dr. West and see if further negotiation regarding authorship credit is possible, or simply accept his mentor's edits. Assuming he decides to discuss authorship with Dr. West, what would be the best way to open this dialogue? Is this a conversation best had in person or would email be more appropriate? If he decides not to say anything, how can he keep his own emotions in check such that it does not sour his relationship with a mentor (and as previously stated, a potential reference)?

5. **Consult as needed.** Malachi should definitely consult with peers, but, as in previous examples, he will need to be cautious in selecting individuals for consultation that will not just tell him what he wants to hear. It would be easy to vent about his concerns with close friends who might support some of his frustrations, but it may be less likely that these friends would offer critical feedback. It would also be important for Malachi to be cautious in consulting with Dr.

West's peers. These individuals may know him well enough to offer key insights, but Malachi should be careful in navigating the political landscape of the academic world.

The Likely Answer

Malachi should probably take a day or two to process his emotions and then reach out to Dr. West to discuss authorship for the paper moving forward.

REPORTING RESULTS (*WHAT SAY WE FOCUS ON THE POSITIVES?*)

Donovan is a supervisor at a drug and alcohol treatment facility. One of his supervisees is Zak, a counselor at the clinic who is also completing his doctorate in counselor education at a local university. As part of his dissertation, Zak has been collecting data from the clinic regarding outcomes of counseling. Donovan was in support of this project, as he hoped to present the data to the clinic's administrators as justification for increased funding. He even teased about these findings at his last meeting with the board of directors, stating that he had "a good student looking at outcome data."

Zak has completed his data analysis and presented the findings in a private meeting with Donovan: Apparently, the aggregate data suggest that attending counseling at this particular treatment facility leads to *increases* in relapse rates. The data appear to be sound, as Zak had several faculty members and colleagues at the university monitoring his work both during data collection and after analysis of the findings.

Needless to say, Donovan is disheartened, but he is also worried about what the board of directors will do when they find out that the clinic and its staff are providing shoddy treatment.

Questions for Discussion

1. *Should Donovan give these findings to the board, or should he wait to review the findings more carefully?*
2. *What about the staff at the clinic? Should Donovan consider withholding results as it might have an impact on their employment?*
3. *Might there be a way to present the results that softens the findings?*

Straight From the Code

1. **G.2.h. Informing Sponsors.** Counselors inform sponsors, institutions, and publication channels regarding research procedures and outcomes. Counselors ensure that appropriate bodies and authorities are given pertinent information and acknowledgment.

2. **G.4.a. Accurate Results.** Counselors plan, conduct, and report research accurately. Counselors do not engage in misleading or fraudulent research, distort data, misrepresent data, or deliberately bias their results. They describe the extent to which results are applicable for diverse populations.

3. **G.4.b. Obligation to Report Unfavorable Results.** Counselors report the results of any research of professional value. Results that reflect unfavorably on institutions, programs, services, prevailing opinions, or vested interests are not withheld.

Applying a Decision-Making Model: Jacob, Roth, Cilento, and Stoler's Model

1. **Recognize the ethical dilemma and be aware of bias hotspots.** Donovan's decision-making in this example is compromised to say the least. He likely feels a sense of attachment to the clinic as well as his employees, and the indication that his work is slipshod in any way is apt to be an uncomfortable revelation for any number of reasons.

2. **Practice mindful awareness.** Because of this, Donovan needs to be very mindful of his actions and the possibility that he could unintentionally veer toward the unethical. Particularly when a personal investment is at stake, counselors need to be very cautious in recognizing whether the decided course of action is actually in the best interest of the profession or whether it simply reflects personal interests masked as something else (à la a Ouija board effect; see Gauchou, Rensink, & Fels, 2012 for a detailed review). In this case, it could be quite easy for Donovan to convince himself he is acting in the best interest of his clinic when in fact he is actually acting in his best interests financially or personally.

3. **Reference the Code of Ethics.** The Code is pretty clear that any results from research conducted need to be presented accurately (G.4.a.), even if they are unfavorable (G.4.b.). The fact that Donovan is aware that sound research was conducted that indicates the clinic is providing poor quality treatment requires acknowledgment. To not do so would be guilt by omission.

4. **Consider alternative options.** Refusing to acknowledge the findings is not an option, and Donovan will likely have no choice but to be honest with the board. Donovan might consider working with Zak to examine the findings more carefully, as the description provided thus far lacks both detail and nuance. Specifically, what factors were assessed and how were they measured? Can the findings be used in some way to better the clinic? Is the outcome of this project a reason to shutter operations or can it instead inform an action plan to improve the quality of services?

5. **Consult as needed.** It would be important for Donovan to consult with a colleague who not only is familiar with research method and design but also has no financial or personal stake in the clinic's success or failure. It would be a good measure of quality to take Zak's findings to an independent researcher at another institution and clarify: What do these results mean exactly? Is there any flaw in the methodology? Does this indicate that the clinic as a whole is inherently problematic, or are there actionable items that can be culled from these findings?

   A consultation with a similar peer, one familiar with methodology and lacking investment in the clinic, would likely be warranted once Donovan begins preparing his presentation of these findings to the board. He will again need to ensure that his dissemination of the results in some way controls for his own biases and the presentation is (for wont of a better term) fair.

The Likely Answer

Donovan should reach out to an independent consultant at a separate university to review the findings, determine how to present this to the board, have someone review his presentation to check for biases, and then present these findings to the board.

RELATIONSHIPS WITH RESEARCH PARTICIPANTS (*QUALITATIVE CASANOVA*)

Daisy is a recently tenured counselor education faculty member at a university. To celebrate her newfound job security, she has decided to study a topic that is of interest to her: the qualitative experiences of clients who have experienced attraction to their counselors. Her project has received approval from the university's institutional review board (IRB), and data collection is underway. She is making use of graduate students to conduct audio-recorded interviews with participants willing to discuss their experiences in counseling and the impact of the attraction.

Daisy just got her first transcribed session from Dylan, one of her grad students who is helping with interviews. The transcript is an hour-long interview of a female undergraduate student (participant X), and based on what Daisy can see in the transcript, Dylan seems to be following the semistructured format as well as the basic interview protocol outlined in the IRB proposal. However, she also notices that the interview contains a great deal more playful banter between Dylan and participant X than she would have expected. Curious, she decides to listen to the audio recording of the interview.

In reviewing the tape, she notes that what reads as playful banter in the transcript sounds more like flirtation on the audio recording. Worse yet, the tape picks up a final 5 minutes of dialogue that Dylan opted not to transcribe, during which he asks participant X out for a coffee date, to which she accepts.

Questions for Discussion

1. *As the interview was over, did Dylan technically do anything wrong?*
2. *How should Daisy handle the situation? Should she speak to Dylan first? Her direct supervisor? Participant X?*
3. *Assuming this does constitute a breach of ethics, what should Daisy do with the data obtained from the interview?*

Straight From the Code

1. **G.3.b. Relationships With Research Participants.** Sexual or romantic counselor–research participant interactions or relationships with current research participants are prohibited. This prohibition applies to both in-person and electronic interactions or relationships.

Applying a Decision-Making Model: Jacob, Roth, Cilento, and Stoler's Model

1. **Recognize the ethical dilemma and be aware of bias hotspots.** It is very likely that Daisy feels a great attachment both to this project and to the data she is attempting to collect. Additionally, her interest in counselor–client boundaries may make her more prone to frustration when witnessing what might be interpreted as the exploitation of a research participant. However, her role as instructor to Dylan might cause her to tread lightly with regard to consequences, as she may view her role as an educator to be more important than her role as an authority figure regarding ethical conduct.

2. **Practice mindful awareness.** As such, Daisy will need to be very cautious in her management of this situation, as her response could potentially lean too far in the direction of retribution (in that she feels angry at Dylan for what he has done) or leniency (in that she feels responsible to train Dylan rather than punish him).

3. **Reference the Code of Ethics.** The Code is decidedly clear that romantic relationships with current participants are completely inappropriate (G.3.b.). What lacks clarity is whether Dylan made romantic overtures during or after completion of the project. During the interview, Daisy noted what could be construed as flirtation, but this interpretation is subjective, and obvious deviations from protocol were not indicated.

   However, the end of the interview does not indicate the end of the project. Qualitative research requires that researchers thoroughly demonstrate trustworthiness in their assessment of the data, and including participants in this process is not uncommon (see Hunt, 2011 for a detailed review). Daisy may need to elicit further information from participant X, and Dylan's behaviors have likely compromised her ability to do so.

4. **Consider alternative options.** It seems obvious that Dylan violated the code of ethics in this case, but how Daisy is to respond is less clear. Her options would be to (a) keep resolution of the matter *in house* by simply informing Dylan this behavior is inappropriate and discarding the data from analysis (this seems an unlikely option, as it negates the severity of Dylan's actions completely) and (b) inform her department chair and/or program director of Dylan's actions and determine what consequences should follow.

5. **Consult as needed.** Daisy might want to consult with another professor in the department before reaching out to her supervisors, but she would need to be cautious in selecting an individual who might help to challenge her perspective. Does this individual know Dylan? Do they have an interest in qualitative research and/or counselor–client boundaries? In what way do they offer a difference of opinion on the matter?

   Regardless, it seems apparent that Daisy should reach out to her supervisors, and potentially the IRB, to ensure transparency of the project and its setbacks. Unless a peer or her department chair has a different perspective to offer, it also seems unlikely that Daisy will be able to use this interview in her study.

The Likely Answer

Daisy needs to meet with Dylan to get more details regarding what happened, consult with a colleague to see if they offer any additional insight, and then present her concerns to her department chair. What consequences Dylan faces will be established in collaboration with the department and/or the university, but the data obtained from this participant should likely not be included in the final analysis. Daisy should also follow up with participant X to discuss the incident and offer additional support as needed.

CONFIDENTIALITY (*WELL…THAT WENT WELL*)

Natasha is a counselor working in quality assurance for a behavioral health insurance provider. A big part of her job is collecting utilization data from members throughout the state to examine trends regarding treatment, types of claims, and anything else that might have an impact on the company's finances.

Today, Natasha has been tasked with presenting her recent data collection efforts to a group of social workers and related administrators from the state's Department of Health and Human Services (DHHS). The presentation is a big deal, and Natasha has been working on her findings for months now. In preparation for this meeting the night before, she sent her PowerPoint slides to the entire group (20 members in total) as well as posted them to a state listserv (400 members in total). Her hope was to disseminate her deidentified findings to the entire state and for attendees at the group either to print and bring these slides to the meeting or to access them via electronic device during the presentation.

Ten minutes in, and the presentation is going well! Despite being nervous, Natasha is presenting all of the information clearly, and the group seems locked in.

Just as Natasha is beginning to feel more comfortable, one of the DHHS members raises their hand. They point out that the slides emailed to the 20 attendees contain Excel charts embedded within. It seems that these charts include names, mental health history, addresses, and social security numbers for thousands of treatment recipients throughout the state.

Questions for Discussion

1. *What should Natasha do in this moment? Stop the presentation? Continue and deal with this information later?*
2. *Regarding this breach of confidentiality, should the treatment recipients be notified?*
3. *How should Natasha's supervisors handle this situation? Should she be reprimanded? If so, to what extent?*

Straight From the Code

1. **G.2.d. Confidentiality of Information.** Information obtained about research participants during the course of research is confidential. Procedures are implemented to protect confidentiality.

2. **G.3.a. Extending Researcher–Participant Boundaries.** Researchers consider the risks and benefits of extending current research relationships beyond conventional parameters. When a nonresearch interaction between the researcher and the research participant may be potentially beneficial, the researcher must document, prior to the interaction (when feasible), the rationale for such an interaction, the potential benefit, and anticipated consequences for the research participant. Such interactions should be initiated with appropriate consent of the research participant. Where unintentional harm occurs to the research participant, the researcher must show evidence of an attempt to remedy such harm.

Applying a Decision-Making Model: Jacob, Roth, Cilento, and Stoler's Model

1. **Recognize the ethical dilemma and be aware of bias hotspots.** With regard to what Natasha should do moving forward, it is likely that her personal biases are related to saving face and not losing her job. As such, she will need to ensure that she is carefully considering the needs of the individuals whose confidence has been betrayed as well as her own need to maintain her job.

2. **Practice mindful awareness.** This will take effort, as it will likely be difficult to consider the needs of these individuals in addition to her job and livelihood, particularly as she faces potential consequences for her actions. She likely feels a great deal of embarrassment about what has happened and may feel the inclination to want to avoid potential repercussions. However, there seem to be few options regarding remediation of this situation that do *not* involve public disclosure regarding what happened.

3. **Reference the Code of Ethics.** Information collected for research purposes is to be kept in confidence (G.2.d.), and researchers must make efforts to remediate when and if harm has occurred (G.3.a.). In this case, confidentiality was clearly breached. If she had only emailed these findings to the meeting attendees, there might be an easier solution to the presenting problem. The posting to the listserv is what makes for the greatest potential concern, as it is unclear to what extent membership is regulated or exactly how many people were granted access to the data. What constitutes remediation in the aftermath of such a violation is unclear, though these individuals will at the very least need to be made aware of what happened in the interest of taking measures to safeguard their identities (i.e., placing a fraud alert on their social security numbers).

4. **Consider alternative options.** In the aftermath of this presentation, Natasha will likely have to find a way to notify these individuals that their personal information has been compromised. In the moment, she has to decide if she should either continue the presentation and notify her supervisor afterward or stop the presentation and notify her supervisor immediately.

   While it is complicated to include the risk of a lawsuit in the process of decision-making, Natasha may want to consider that all of her behaviors from this point forward may be the subject of intense scrutiny (particularly if one of these individuals sues for some reason). While there may be little that can be practically done in the moment, her concern for these individuals may be better represented by immediately stopping the presentation rather than continuing after having found out about a major violation of confidentiality.

5. **Consult as needed.** As in many cases of ethical decision-making, Natasha does not have the option to consult with a peer (unless colleagues are present, or her supervisor is unavailable). As such, the best option may be to forego peer consultation at this time in favor of discussing the matter with her direct supervisor.

The Likely Answer

Natasha needs to take a deep breath, thank this individual for pointing this out, and then inform the rest of the group that a break will take place while she consults with her supervisor. Afterward, members should be notified via email or regular post to make them aware that a data breach has occurred.

CLIENT PARTICIPATION (*A B D...EASY AS 1, 2, 3*)

Diamanda is a part-time doctoral student in counselor education at a large research university. She has just been approved to begin data collection for her dissertation project: a survey of transgender adolescents. The estimated sample size necessary to complete her study and satisfy her power requirements is ambitious, as she needs to recruit no fewer than 189 transgender adolescents to take part in a 20-minute survey that can be completed online.

After 4 weeks of effort, Diamanda is about 100 participants short and has exhausted the majority of her available resources. Despite having posted a link to her survey on just about every listserv related to her topic she can find (and having posted on multiple occasions in several cases), she is running out of options regarding potential participants.

She does have one available outlet, though: her clients. In addition to her part-time status as a doctoral student, she is a full-time director of a counseling center in a large metropolitan area that works exclusively with LGBTQ youth.

Questions for Discussion

1. *Is it acceptable for Diamanda to use her own clients for research?*
2. *Would it be possible for Diamanda to be certain that these clients are participating of their own volition and not out of loyalty to their counselor?*
3. *If she did use her own clients as participants, how will she notate this in her write-up?*

Straight From the Code

1. **G.2.c. Client Participation.** Counselors conducting research involving clients make clear in the informed consent process that clients are

free to choose whether to participate in research activities. Counselors take necessary precautions to protect clients from adverse consequences of declining or withdrawing from participation.

Applying a Decision-Making Model: Jacob, Roth, Cilento, and Stoler's Model

1. **Recognize the ethical dilemma and be aware of bias hotspots.** The most pressing bias that Diamanda faces here is pressure to complete her dissertation. The process of completing a dissertation is strenuous to say the least (Flynn, Chasek, Harper, Murphy, & Jorgensen, 2012), and it is safe to assume from the description that Diamanda is feeling pressure to put this project behind her. Not completing this project is likely holding her back from either a more satisfying career or a potential salary increase at her current position as a function of a change in education status.

2. **Practice mindful awareness.** As she has a lot of "skin in the game," Diamanda needs to be very careful that her efforts are directed toward the best interest of her clients. This will indeed be challenging, as she might argue that her project and its findings are an asset to the transgender population she serves. However, she should also carefully examine the experience from her clients' perspective: Being solicited for research by a treating clinician will likely feel coercive if not presented appropriately.

3. **Reference the Code of Ethics.** Thankfully for Diamanda, the Code does not specifically preclude counselors from using their clients as participants in research projects. It does, however, state that necessary precautions need to be taken to ensure that clients are choosing to participate of their own volition and that they feel confident that they will face no adverse consequences if they decline.

   As such, Diamanda could find recourse to recruit clients for her study, but specific protocol would need to be followed. First, she would have to obtain approval from both her dissertation committee (or her chair at least) and her university's IRB for research. Assuming this is not a problem, she will next have to make certain that participants are de-identified such that she as the research/director is unaware of participant identity. As her project is an anonymous survey, this will likely prove easier than if she were attempting to conduct a qualitative inquiry. Any incentives for participation will likely have to be managed by an individual other than Diamanda; for example, if participants receive an email gift card for their participation, she will have to make sure that someone other than herself collects participant emails to distribute awards.

4. **Consider alternative options.** Though the Code does allow for research conducted using clients, Diamanda might consider simply

working harder to find participants outside of her place of employment. The aforementioned process will likely be enough to safeguard client confidentiality, but the degree to which clients feel safe to refuse would be more challenging to assess. Additionally, Diamanda, particularly in her role as director, has now set a precedent such that research and collection of data by staff members for the purpose of completing a degree is now acceptable. This is particularly problematic if it clashes with the center's purpose or mission.

5. **Consult with peers as needed.** Diamanda's first consultation should be with her dissertation chair, though she might also want to consult with other administrative personnel at the center.

The Likely Answer

Diamanda should first consult with her dissertation chair, relevant administration at the center, and her university's IRB to discuss her plans. If all are in agreement that her procedures are sound (and client confidence can be ensured), she may have recourse to pull from her center's clients.

PRECAUTIONS TO AVOID INJURY (*CAN WE TALK ABOUT THIS A LITTLE MORE?*)

Ian is a tenure-track faculty member in a counselor education program at a private Catholic university. As scholarly productivity is a valued part of the tenure process, he is putting together a follow-up to some of his previous research regarding the treatment of bipolar disorder. His previous paper had examined aggregate data regarding suicide attempts among individuals meeting the criteria for bipolar disorder; his next piece of research is going to be a qualitative inquiry of individual experiences with suicidal thoughts, again with individuals meeting the criteria for bipolar disorder.

After presenting his study outline to the university's IRB, Ian's project is rejected outright. The board claims it will not support his research for fear that discussing suicide with a population of individuals struggling with a "serious mental health disorder" may trigger emotional distress or increase the likelihood of an attempt.

Questions for Discussion

1. *Is the board correct in their assumption? Would discussing suicide with this population put them at greater risk for a future suicide attempt or further emotional distress?*
2. *What would be the best way for Ian to respond to these concerns?*
3. *Is there an alternate research design that would not only allow Ian to complete his research but also mollify the board's concerns?*

Straight From the Code

1. **G.1.e. Precautions to Avoid Injury.** Counselors who conduct research are responsible for their participants' welfare throughout the research process and should take reasonable precautions to avoid causing emotional, physical, or social harm to participants.

Applying a Decision-Making Model: Jacob, Roth, Cilento, and Stoler's Model

1. **Recognize the ethical dilemma and be aware of bias hotspots.** As in the previous case, the most pressing bias that Ian faces here is pressure to complete his research. The pressure for faculty, particularly junior faculty such as Ian, can be tremendous indeed (Grimes et al., 2018).

2. **Practice mindful awareness.** Ian should carefully consider his own internal experiences related to managing the gravity of his current position. In this case, Ian will have to be certain that he does not favor the needs of his research over the needs of his participants.

   Ian should also practice mindful awareness in his interactions with the IRB as he moves forward in this process. Collegiality is critical in the world of academia, and Ian might be offended by the outright rejection of his proposal as well as the board's illness-focused language (e.g., "serious mental health disorders"). He will need to do his best to have empathy for the members of the IRB, as they are likely acting out of unfamiliarity rather than malice.

3. **Reference the Code of Ethics.** The Code is clear that counselors take necessary steps to keep research participants out of harm's way. However, it is unclear what specific concerns held by the IRB are with merit, as current research does not appear to support their concerns. Ian's study requires participants to discuss their experiences with suicidal ideation; though review boards often worry, there is limited empirical support for the idea that talking about suicide increases the likelihood of an attempt for any population (Dazzi, Gribble, Wessely, & Fear, 2014). As such, he has recourse to respond to the board with his concerns and request that they reconsider the decision not to support his project.

   However, Ian will have to make certain that he provides his participants with necessary support if they should become triggered in any way by any of the project-specific inquiries. This could include a list of local or national crisis support services, though the specifics of these requirements would likely have to be negotiated with the IRB.

4. **Consider alternative options.** Though there is limited evidence to support the IRB's concerns, Ian might consider looking into alternative

methods for his project. For example, would the IRB (and his research) be better served if the project were a quantitative measure that has research to support its efficacy?

5. **Consult as needed.** As Ian is a new faculty, he might begin by consulting with peers at the university to better understand the concerns and nuances of the IRB. This might in part be an inquiry into university politics, but he should at the very least be aware of the board's composition—are any members affiliated with the mental health profession such that they are aware of the aforementioned research regarding discussion of suicide and the impact on attempts?

The Likely Answer

Ian should first consult with peers to better understand the board's composition and expertise. Following a careful review of their feedback, he should provide a response that educates them regarding their trepidations and request further dialogue to help improve the study overall.

IN-CLASS DISCUSSION AND EXERCISES

Group Discussion: Confidentiality Revisited

Though confidentiality is critical to counseling, the utilization of quality assurance measures adds a layer of complexity. While not all counselors are required to conduct research, making certain to collect outcome measures to explore the efficacy of intervention is strongly recommended, which often times requires collecting personal or sensitive client data.

In your current (or future) practice setting, what types of quality assurance measures are being utilized (or would make the most sense to utilize)? Measures of depression? Substance abuse recidivism? In collecting these data, what types of security measures are (or should be) in place?

Group Discussion: Empathy Revisited

Imagine you are a client in psychotherapy, and you just received a notice from your insurance company that your social security number and treatment history may have been accidentally disseminated in a public forum. How would you feel about this? How might you respond? What, if anything, could the insurance company do to remedy this situation?

Role Play: Well...That Went Well

Using the scenario described in *Well...That Went Well*, role-play possible outcomes. Have one member play the role of Natasha and another play the role of her supervisor when they meet to discuss the situation at hand. If you were Natasha, how might you begin a dialogue? As her supervisor, how might you actually feel or respond in the moment after one of your supervisees discloses a mistake this egregious?

Documentation: Problem, Data, Assessment, and Plan

Using the Problem, Data, Assessment, and Plan (PDAP) format, pick one of the cases and write a progress note indicating the following:

Problem: What were the presenting concerns of this particular interaction?

Data: What, objectively, has happened? Remember to write this without subjective language or interpretation.

Assessment: As the counselor or supervisor in question, what *should* be done? Be sure to demonstrate comprehensive use of the decision-making model in this section.

Plan: What *will* be done? Be sure to outline a comprehensive plan that relates to the decision-making model.

References

Dazzi, T., Gribble, R., Wessely, S., & Fear, N. T. (2014). Does asking about suicide and related behaviours induce suicidal ideation? What is the evidence? *Psychological Medicine, 44*(16), 3361–3363. doi:10.1017/S0033291714001299

Flynn, S. V., Chasek, C. L., Harper, I. F., Murphy, K. M., & Jorgensen, M. F. (2012). A qualitative inquiry of the counseling dissertation process. *Counselor Education and Supervision, 51*(4), 242–255. doi:10.1002/j.1556-6978.2012.00018.x

Garcia, J. G., Cartwright, B., Winston, S. M., & Borzuchowska, B. (2003). A transcultural integrative model for ethical decision-making in counseling. *Journal of Counseling and Development, 81*(3), 268–277. doi:10.1002/j.1556-6678.2003.tb00253.x

Gauchou, H. L., Rensink, R. A., & Fels, S. (2012). Expression of nonconscious knowledge via ideomotor actions. *Consciousness and Cognition, 21*(2), 976–982. doi:10.1016/j.concog.2012.01.016

Grimes, D. R., Bauch, C. T., & Ioannidis, J. P. (2018). Modelling science trustworthiness under publish or perish pressure. *Royal Society Open Science, 5*(1), 171511. doi:10.1098/rsos.171511

Hunt, B. (2011). Publishing qualitative research in counseling journals. *Journal of Counseling and Development, 89*(3), 296–300. doi:10.1002/j.1556-6678.2011.tb00092.x

Jacob, C. J., Roth, G., Cilento, B., & Stoler, J. (2015). The 2014 ACA code of ethics: What's new, what's the same, and what matters for practicing counselors. *Journal of the Pennsylvania Counseling Association, 14*, 39–46.

CHAPTER 8

DISTANCE COUNSELING, TECHNOLOGY, AND SOCIAL MEDIA (SECTION H OF THE ACA CODE OF ETHICS)

INTRODUCTION

Surprisingly, a section devoted to technology was not added to the American Counseling Association (ACA) Code of Ethics until its most recent revision in 2014. The benefits and detriments of increased utility of technology are unavoidable in all professions, and counseling is no exception. The cases in this section highlight the ways in which technological advancements have made counseling both easier and more complicated.

All cases will be assessed using Kocet and Herlihy's counselor's value-based conflict model (CVCM; 2014) for making an ethical decision.

COUNSELOR'S VALUE-BASED CONFLICT MODEL APPROACH (KOCET & HERLIHY, 2014)

Kocet and Herlihy developed the CVCM (2014) as a way for counselors to work through personal values while maintaining boundaries and abiding by the 2014 ACA Code of Ethics. The CVCM should not be considered a stand-alone model but one that complements other models in the ethical decision-making process. This model is a direct response to multiple legal cases where counselors' values were challenged, most specifically addressing the 2014 ACA Code of Ethics, A.11.b Values Within Termination and Referral. Steps in the model include the following:

1. **Determine the nature of the value-based conflict.** What specific values or beliefs of the client(s), the profession, and the counselor(s) involved are at play?

2. **Explore core issues and potential barriers to providing appropriate standard of care.** What are the practical or abstract obstacles in reaching a resolution?

3. **Seek assistance/remediation for providing appropriate standard of care.** Consult with peers or supervisors as needed.

4. **Determine and evaluate possible courses of action.** Develop a list of possible resolutions, and carefully consider their potential outcomes.
5. **Ensure that proposed actions promote client welfare.** In considering their potential outcomes, determine which resolutions will best promote the well-being of clients.

USE OF PUBLIC SOCIAL MEDIA: PART 1 (*METAL HEALTH WILL DRIVE YOU MAD!*)

Kat is a counselor and clinical supervisor working for a community mental health center. Her time is split between seeing clients struggling with myriad mental health concerns and supervising a staff of eight master's level counselors. The center is sponsored by a local Catholic university, and faith-based values are included in the mission statement.

During her lunch hour, Kat is perusing her social media pages. In looking through a "people you might know" suggestion, she notices that one of her supervisees—Maureen, a recently licensed counselor in her mid-20s—has a publicly available page. Curious, she clicks on the page and scrolls through some of her pictures.

Kat is quite surprised by the content. It appears that Maureen has a strong interest in what could best be described as *heavy metal*. Many of the pictures are of Maureen and her friends drinking at concerts featuring bands with names such as *Mayhem*, *Full of Hell*, and *The Body*. After conducting a quick search on the Internet, Kat discovers that many of these bands espouse satanic imagery as part of their aesthetic. To wit, some of the pictures on Maureen's page show the bands' stage setups including pentagrams and inverted crosses.

Questions for Discussion

1. *As this is not Kat's social media page, is she obligated to do anything about this? Was it an invasion of privacy to look through Maureen's pictures without her permission?*
2. *As she is employed by a Catholic institution, is Kat obligated to report these findings to any of her supervisors?*
3. *How might Kat prevent something like this from happening again in the future?*

Straight From the Code

1. **H.6.a. Virtual Professional Presence.** In cases where counselors wish to maintain a professional and personal presence for social media use, separate professional and personal web pages and profiles are created to clearly distinguish between the two kinds of virtual presence.

2. **H.6.d. Use of Public Social Media.** Counselors take precautions to avoid disclosing confidential information through public social media.

Applying a Decision-Making Model: Kocet and Herlihy's CVCM (2014)

1. **Determine the nature of the value-based conflict.** In this case, no specific ethical code according to the counselor profession has been violated, though Maureen should have worked more diligently to separate her personal and professional Internet presence (H.6.a.). Maureen is free to appreciate whatever art or music she prefers, but the values and ethics of the institution that employs her are independent of the ACA. In this case, Maureen's personal interests are clearly at odds with the institution, and her supervisor (Kat) is now aware of this.

2. **Explore core issues and potential barriers to providing appropriate standard of care.** While it has been established that counselors can be dismissed from the profession for values that conflict with the ACA's (Herlihy, Herman, & Greden, 2014; Kaplan, 2014), Maureen has not expressed any specific values that directly conflict those of the counseling profession. However, while religious institutions are beholden to refraining from discrimination as a function of Title IX of the Education Amendments Act of 1972 (2019), they are free to discriminate based on religion. As such, the school might have cause for action if they were to discover that Maureen's values were not in keeping with the mission of the university.

3. **Seek assistance/remediation for providing appropriate standard of care.** Kat might want to first process this concern with a peer separate from the institution, though the intention would be less to gain a specific answer and more to make sense of her own biases and concerns before deciding how to respond. If she holds (or does not hold) strong religious values of her own, this might influence her response. Specifically, if she identifies as more secular than Catholic, she may be remiss to respond despite the fact that Kat's values are not in step with the university's mission. However, if she identifies strongly with the Catholic faith, she may be more harsh or punitive in her response to these findings than is warranted.

4. **Determine and evaluate possible courses of action.** One option would be to ignore these images and say nothing. However, this could become problematic if one of the center's clients stumbles across these pictures the same way that Maureen did. Another option would be to simply ask Kat to remove these photos and keep the response *in house*, though Maureen could be seen as complicit if the university found out

that this occurred, and they were not informed. A final option would be for Maureen to first ask that Kat remove these images followed by consultation with her supervisors to clarify institutional policies. It may be that the university has a zero-tolerance policy for value-based conflicts, but there may already be an established precedent for handling concerns such as these.

5. **Ensure that proposed actions promote client welfare.** The extent to which Maureen's taste in art and music has an effect on her clients' well-being is questionable, though the impact may be perceived as harmful by the institution. It has also not been established to what extent Maureen allows her personal values to affect her work. Specifically, does she disparage Catholic values in her work with her clients? Does she regularly discuss her interests as part of her clinical work in any capacity? Does she have a demonstrated record of keeping her professional and private interests separate?

The Likely Answer

Maureen should first ask that Kat remove these images and then speak with her supervisors to clarify institutional policies.

USE OF PUBLIC SOCIAL MEDIA: PART 2 (*SIX DEGREES OF SEPARATION*)

Brendan is a counselor in private practice where he sees about 30 clients a week. His partner, Gordon, is a photographer in the same area, where he has won several regional awards for his work as a family photographer. As part of Gordon's business, he has a social media page that includes samples of his work. Many of the sample photographs are of Brendan, their two dogs, and the regular trips and vacations they have taken together. Brendan is a private person and admittedly camera shy, but he agreed to allow the pictures posted to social media as it was necessary for Gordon's business.

During a counseling session with Angela, a client who has a history of struggling with boundaries, she casually mentions following Gordon's social media page. She even makes a comment about how "cute" Gordon is and how "adorable" their dogs are.

Questions for Discussion

1. *As this is not Brendan's social media page, is he obligated to do anything about this?*
2. *If Brendan feels uncomfortable with this, should he ask Gordon to "unfollow" Angela? Should he ask Angela to "unfollow" Gordon?*
3. *How might Brendan prevent something like this from happening again in the future?*

Straight From the Code

1. **H.6.a. Virtual Professional Presence.** In cases where counselors wish to maintain a professional and personal presence for social media use, separate professional and personal web pages and profiles are created to clearly distinguish between the two kinds of virtual presence.

2. **H.6.d. Use of Public Social Media.** Counselors take precautions to avoid disclosing confidential information through public social media.

Applying a Decision-Making Model: Kocet and Herlihy's CVCM (2014)

1. **Determine the nature of the value-based conflict.** In this case, no specific ethical code has been violated. Instead, the main concern is that Brendan values his privacy and is likely uncomfortable with a client (Angela or otherwise) having a direct line to his personal life. However, this is a public social media page, and Angela is well within her right to follow whomever she wants. Additionally, asking Gordon to remove her from his followers will identify her as a client and violate her confidentiality.

2. **Explore core issues and potential barriers to providing appropriate standard of care.** Brendan may need to carefully examine his own biases as far as his decision-making process is concerned. Though he is a private person by nature, neither Angela nor Gordon behaved inappropriately in this context. The core concern is likely that Brendan feels uncomfortable with the amount of personal information his clients have access to.

   Additionally, the Code only states that counselors take precautions to avoid disclosing client information (H.6.d.) and that counselors distinguish between their personal and professional social media pages (H.6.a.). Nothing is directly stated about the social media presence of a partner or social contact.

3. **Seek assistance/remediation for providing appropriate standard of care.** Brendan might want to first process this concern in supervision, though the intention would be less to gain a specific answer from his supervisor and more to make sense of his own biases and concerns before he responds. It may be that he feels so strongly about his need for privacy that he may be too quick to push for an answer that may ask too much of those involved (e.g., asking Gordon to delete his social media page completely).

4. **Determine and evaluate possible courses of action.** One option would be to ask Gordon to remove Angela from his list of followers.

However, this would identify Angela as a client and betray her confidentiality. Another option would be to ask Angela to no longer follow Gordon's social media page, though he has no authority to enforce this (i.e., Angela has autonomy and cannot be forced to do so). A final option would be to ask Gordon to remove all of Brendan's personal pictures from his social media page.

5. **Ensure that proposed actions promote client welfare.** Instead of telling her to *unfollow* Gordon, Brendan might simply ask Angela to do so, thus keeping her autonomy in place. The difference between asking and telling may seem inconsequential, but it is important to remember that (a) Angela did not do anything *wrong* in this case and that (b) autonomy is a core ethical principle. If she is unwilling to do so for some reason, this is her choice. Additionally, Brendan will need to be sure that his request does not come across as unintentionally coercive, in that his asking her is actually received by Angela as a directive.

   Asking Gordon to remove Brendan's personal photographs may be a reasonable option as well, particularly if Brendan wants to avoid situations like this in the future. Social media presence can be difficult to regulate, but this may be an obvious option if this level of publicly available personal information makes him uncomfortable.

The Likely Answer

Brendan should ask Angela if she is willing to unfollow Gordon and then ask Gordon to remove any personal images of Brendan from his public social media pages.

CLIENT VIRTUAL PRESENCE (*SOMETIMES IT FEELS LIKE SOMEBODY'S WATCHING ME*)

Chip is a counselor in private practice where he has been seeing Lee, a young man in his 20s struggling with opiate addiction, for individual counseling. Sessions have been weekly for the past 3 months, and Lee reports to have remained sober for the duration.

Chip, however, is suspicious of some of the claims Lee makes during these sessions. For example, despite arriving for sessions in a beat-up Geo Prism, Lee insists that he is "basically a multimillionaire" as a result of his successful recording company. All the sober coping skills and future plans discussed in session seem to revolve around this company, in that Lee states that he identifies with the work and plans to use the money from the company to support himself in perpetuity.

Chip is worried that Lee is fabricating these stories, either to impress him or as a way of avoiding the dire nature of his current predicament. In addition to noting the condition of his car, Chip notes that Lee rarely changes his clothes. All told, his hygiene indicates that he may be living out of his Geo.

Chip has made several attempts to question the "plot holes" in Lee's story, but to no avail; Lee is just unwilling to offer any indication that his story of a multimillion dollar recording empire is anything but completely true.

As a last resort, Chip is considering conducting an Internet search to verify the accuracy of Lee's claims. He reasons that if there is any truth to his story, a simple Google search should be able to confirm or deny everything.

Questions for Discussion

1. *Is an Internet search appropriate in this case as it has to do less with curiosity on behalf of the counselor and more to do with aiding in the client's treatment?*
2. *Is there another way to verify Lee's claims?*
3. *Is it really Chip's job to play detective and verify the accuracy of Lee's claims?*

Straight From the Code

1. **H.6.c. Client Virtual Presence.** Counselors respect the privacy of their clients' presence on social media unless given consent to view such information.

Applying a Decision-Making Model: Kocet and Herlihy's CVCM (2014)

1. **Determine the nature of the value-based conflict.** The concern is that Chip very much wants to help Lee in planning his future, but he is worried that Lee is approaching these concerns in a manner that is both reckless and unrealistic. However, the Code is clear that counselors respect the privacy of their clients regarding Internet searches unless they are given permission to do so. Therein lies the crux of the problem presented: Chip is not hoping to find personal information about his client out of idle curiosity. Instead, he is concerned that a client's treatment is being severely compromised due to embarrassment or some other propensity that has not been explored.

2. **Explore core issues and potential barriers to providing appropriate standard of care.** Clients deserve privacy, and the goal of the counselor is not to act as a private investigator. If Lee is unwilling to discuss the nature of his current predicament, this is his choice. Per the basics of motivational interviewing (Miller & Rollnick, 2013), Chip is unlikely to gain much traction in his efforts to help Lee if Lee is unwilling to do so.

3. **Seek assistance/remediation for providing appropriate standard of care.** As with the previous cases in this chapter, Chip might want to first process this concern in supervision. Once more, the intention would be less to gain a specific answer from his supervisor and more to make sense of his own biases and concerns before he responds. Is he genuinely concerned for Lee's well-being, or is he more irritated with Lee's denial of reality?

4. **Determine and evaluate possible courses of action.** It would be plausible to simply refrain from challenging Lee's assertions about his wealth as this is what he is willing to discuss in counseling for the time being. However, this runs the risk of ignoring the severity of Lee's current predicament and not allowing him to get the help and support he needs to succeed. Chip could also conduct a very simple Internet search to verify the accuracy of Lee's claims in the hopes that this would *back him into a corner*, such that Lee would have no choice but to address his current predicament directly. Finally, Chip could simply keep the door open for further exploration of Lee's presenting concerns and make efforts to offer Lee reflection and insight as appropriate.

5. **Ensure that proposed actions promote client welfare.** Unfortunately, none of the presenting options are ideal. If Chip refrains from addressing the discrepancies in Lee's story, he is technically abiding by the Code of Ethics' requirement regarding Internet privacy. However, he may be missing an opportunity to help Lee confront his problem more directly and establish more realistic sober supports and coping skills. If he does play *Internet detective* and attempts to confront Lee with the inconsistencies of his report, he is technically violating an ethical principle and likely damaging rapport with his client.

The Likely Answer

Chip should not search his clients using the Internet without their permission. He should do his best to provide Lee with support and compassion, and work with him in session to determine the feasibility of specific plans and related coping skills.

DISTANCE COUNSELING USING ELECTRONIC MEDIA (*WAIT, WHAT TIME IS IT?*)

Mike is a counselor in private practice. In keeping with the times, he regularly texts and emails with his clients for scheduling purposes. He has outlined in the consent form that texts and emails are only for scheduling purposes and discusses this during the intake session with all of his clients. Additionally, his informed consent form refers clients to a crisis support line if they require help outside of business hours.

One of Mike's clients, Elle, has been seeing Mike for the past year for depression. She has a history of suicide attempts and struggles regularly with depressive episodes connected to her marriage. She works as a nurse for a local hospital, so her schedule varies tremendously, and she is rarely available to talk on the phone during regular business hours. As such, her appointments with Mike are almost always arranged via text or email. This arrangement has worked well for both, though Mike has made it clear with her on several occasions the importance of boundaries where these communications are concerned.

Tonight, Mike is awakened suddenly at 3 a.m. by a text from Elle. Bleary eyed and half awake, he reads the message that only states "Can we talk? I'm thinking of killing myself."

Questions for Discussion

1. *How should Mike respond in the moment? Since he has made clear the boundaries related to text messages, is he obligated to respond at all?*
2. *Is there anything Mike could have done to have prevented this from happening in the first place?*
3. *If Mike had received this as a voicemail to his practice the next day, would that have been better?*

Straight From the Code

1. **H.1.b. Laws and Statutes.** Counselors who engage in the use of distance counseling, technology, and social media within their counseling practice understand that they may be subject to laws and regulations of both the counselor's practicing location and the client's place of residence. Counselors ensure that their clients are aware of pertinent legal rights and limitations governing the practice of counseling across state lines or international boundaries.

2. **H.4.b. Professional Boundaries in Distance Counseling.** Counselors understand the necessity of maintaining a professional relationship with their clients. Counselors discuss and establish professional boundaries with clients regarding the appropriate use and/or application of technology and the limitations of its use within the counseling relationship (e.g., lack of confidentiality, times when not appropriate to use).

3. **H.4.f. Communication Differences in Electronic Media.** Counselors consider the differences between face-to-face and electronic communication (nonverbal and verbal cues) and how these may affect the counseling process. Counselors educate clients on how to prevent and address potential misunderstandings arising from the lack of visual cues and voice intonations when communicating electronically.

Applying a Decision-Making Model: Kocet and Herlihy's CVCM (2014)

1. **Determine the nature of the value-based conflict.** Mike had not planned on providing distance counseling, but he appears to have stumbled his way into it. Despite having outlined the intended limits of electronic communications both in writing and in person, Elle has pushed against the outlined boundaries and expressed a serious mental health concern via text. If Mike does not respond, he is denying Elle support during a time of pretty serious need (and to a client with a history of suicide attempts). If he responds via text, he is engaging in a form of treatment that he has indicated, both in his consent form and in discussions, that he is inexpert at providing.

   Regardless of these problems, the primary concern is making sure that Elle gets the help and support that she needs in this moment.

2. **Explore core issues and potential barriers to providing appropriate standard of care.** It is not uncommon for text-based counseling to occur, and some preliminary research has suggested positive outcomes (Nesmith, 2018). However, Mike has indicated no established structure for providing these services as well as indicating that this is not a standard component of his practice. As such, responding via text is likely not appropriate, but simply referring Elle to the emergency crisis line seems ineffectual as well.

3. **Seek assistance/remediation for providing appropriate standard of care.** At this hour, it is unlikely that Mike will have options to reach out to a peer or supervisor. He may reach out to crisis services in his area to ask that a well check (a visit to the client's home by crisis services) take place, but it is probably not advisable to initiate this without further query.

4. **Determine and evaluate possible courses of action.** One option would be to text back, but this again opens Mike to the possibility of engaging in an area of practice that is outside his scope of practice. He might call back and check in with Elle to determine if crisis services should conduct a well check, though this is clearly a violation of client–counselor boundaries.

5. **Ensure that proposed actions promote client welfare.** In this case, a bending of client–counselor boundaries seems the only reasonable solution. Not responding is not an option, though any response—that is, responding to a client text at 3 a.m. when this is not an established method of practice—will likely constitute an overstep of established boundaries. Mike's only hope might be to allow for an exception in this case and make clear with Elle what appropriate boundaries are moving forward.

The Likely Answer

Mike should call Elle back, provide brief support via telephone, determine if crisis services should be called, and discuss appropriate boundaries with Elle during their next meeting.

COMMUNICATION DIFFERENCES AND EFFECTIVENESS OF SERVICES (*I CAN'T HEAR YOU! I THINK WE MIGHT BE BREAKING UP*)

Nasir is a counselor in private practice. One of his clients—Andrea, whom he has been seeing steadily for depression over the past 2 years—has just announced that she is relocating for work to a different state. She has indicated reluctance to begin seeing a new counselor and has asked Nasir if he would be willing to meet for videoconference counseling sessions instead.

Nasir has no experience using videoconferencing, but he trusts that Andrea's request is valid, particularly as he is the only counselor out of the seven she has seen in the past 3 years that she stayed with for more than one session. Based on this as well as her history of success in managing her depression since they began counseling, Nasir agrees to see her using a videoconferencing software program. He is unable to bill through Andrea's insurance for these services and instead charges the standard rate for outpatient counseling that Andrea pays out of pocket.

Three sessions of video counseling later, Nasir is struggling. The Internet connection at his office has never been great, and his sessions with Andrea are regularly interrupted by technical difficulties requiring him to stop the session, restart the videoconferencing software, and reconnect with Andrea. At times, there is a delay or a freeze, during which Nasir can hear Andrea but cannot see her.

At the end of this third session, Nasir checks in with Andrea to ask her how she feels about their current treatment structure. Her response is "Well, it's better than having to switch counselors, I guess."

Questions for Discussion

1. *Is it up to Nasir or Andrea to determine if this particular treatment approach is effective?*
2. *Should Nasir have agreed to this arrangement in the first place if he lacked the resources and expertise to do so?*
3. *Should Nasir continue treating Andrea? If so, what steps would be reasonable for him to take to ensure that services are as effective as possible?*

Straight From the Code

1. **H.4.d. Effectiveness of Services.** When distance counseling services are deemed ineffective by the counselor or client, counselors consider

delivering services face-to-face. If the counselor is not able to provide face-to-face services (e.g., lives in another state), the counselor assists the client in identifying appropriate services.

2. **H.4.f. Communication Differences in Electronic Media.** Counselors consider the differences between face-to-face and electronic communication (nonverbal and verbal cues) and how these may affect the counseling process. Counselors educate clients on how to prevent and address potential misunderstandings arising from the lack of visual cues and voice intonations when communicating electronically.

Applying a Decision-Making Model: Kocet and Herlihy's CVCM (2014)

1. **Determine the nature of the value-based conflict.** It is hard to say whether continuing treatment in this fashion is in the best interest of Andrea or not. On one hand, it may be appropriate given her reported difficulties both with depression and with connecting to counselors, in general (not to mention the stress of her recent transition). On the other, Nasir may have convinced himself that he is the only/best option regarding Andrea's continued treatment.

   Regardless, the concern now is that services provided are substandard. Nasir must decide whether to continue treating Andrea (and find a way to improve the quality of services provided) or to simply help Andrea transition to a new counselor (despite her reported desire *not* to do so).

2. **Explore core issues and potential barriers to providing appropriate standard of care.** The utility of *online counseling* and its ethical concerns has been a focus for some time now (e.g., Shaw & Shaw, 2006). At present, standards for what constitutes successful online services have yet to be determined, though the American Psychological Association has indicated that the clinician needs to be licensed in the state where the client is being treated (2019) and the ACA has clarified that many states require clinicians to be licensed in the state in which the client is receiving services (Kaplan & Matz, 2014). In general, the consensus seems to be that while online services are not ideal, they are reasonable in situations where the client would be unable to obtain services in some other fashion (Remley & Herlihy, 2019).

   In this case, it seems that there is no indication that Andrea would be incapable of receiving services otherwise; just that she prefers meeting with Nasir in this substandard fashion instead of seeking support from a different counselor. The concern is that Nasir is operating outside of his scope of competence (e.g., video-based counseling is not an area of identified competency), and he has concerns that the services provided are not in his client's best interest.

3. **Seek assistance/remediation for providing appropriate standard of care.** In addition to reaching out to his direct supervisor, Nasir might try to consult with other clinicians in his area who provide video-based counseling services to determine if there are any practical changes he can make to his software or related technology that might improve service delivery.

   However, the concern about providing services to a client out of state may make this a nonissue. Nasir should clarify what the state laws are in Andrea's state (as well as his own) regarding whether it is appropriate to continue with these services at all.

4. **Determine and evaluate possible courses of action.** Assuming state laws allow him to continue with this practice, one option would be to continue treating Andrea but obtain additional training in distance counseling and find a way to improve quality of services provided (e.g., improve his hardware, software, or Internet service such that gaps in exchanges and interactions are less common). Another option would be to simply help Andrea transition to a new counselor in her area.

5. **Ensure that proposed actions promote client welfare.** Assuming that state laws permit it, Nasir could certainly make use of his clinical acumen to determine if continuing with improved technology and additional training would be enough to warrant continued treatment in this fashion. However, it would be very important for him to consult with his supervisor or other trusted colleagues to ensure that others see this as the most viable option as well. Again, Andrea may be in the best care with Nasir, but she may also need assistance with letting go of her connection to Nasir and beginning a relationship with a therapist in her area.

The Likely Answer

Nasir should first check to see if state law (both his state and hers) permits distance counseling. Assuming yes, he may have the option to continue counseling with her if he deems it clinically necessary and he can improve the quality of services provided.

CLIENT VERIFICATION (*IS IT REALLY YOU?*)

Shanta is a licensed professional counselor who provides most of her clinical services through distance counseling. During and throughout the process, Shanta always verifies that her clients are who they say they are. As an extra step, Shanta has each client text a code word that is created by the client to her 5 minutes before sessions begin.

Last week, one of Shanta's clients, Teresa, shared that her husband has accused her of cheating and was insistent that Teresa provide him with all of her passwords and logins for her social media, email, and cell phone. Teresa says that she obliged his request out of fear but that she also shared her login and password information to this counseling account. To account for this, they agree to change the code word used to initiate sessions.

Shanta receives a text 3 hours after the session ostensibly from Teresa, confirming their next appointment. However, despite the fact that the code word used is correct, Shanta notes the messages sent are inconsistent with Teresa's normal tone. She becomes suspicious that the texts are actually coming from Teresa's husband when "Teresa" asks if Shanta can remind her about what was discussed during their past session.

Questions for Discussion

1. *Is the use of a pass code ironclad? Specifically, should Shanta make assumptions about identity if all appropriate protocols have been met?*
2. *If she chooses not to provide information, should she express her concerns that "Teresa" is not who she claims to be over text?*
3. *How should Shanta address this during her next session with Teresa?*

Straight From the Code

1. **H.3. Client Verification.** Counselors who engage in the use of distance counseling, technology, and/or social media to interact with clients take steps to verify the client's identity at the beginning and throughout the therapeutic process. Verification can include, but is not limited to, using code words, numbers, graphics, or other nondescript identifiers.

2. **H.4.b. Professional Boundaries in Distance Counseling.** Counselors understand the necessity of maintaining a professional relationship with their clients. Counselors discuss and establish professional boundaries with clients regarding the appropriate use and/or application of technology and the limitations of its use within the counseling relationship (e.g., lack of confidentiality, times when not appropriate to use).

Applying a Decision-Making Model: Kocet and Herlihy's CVCM (2014)

1. **Determine the nature of the value-based conflict.** The concern here is less connected to value than it is to instinct, as Shanta technically has no reason not to believe "Teresa" in this case, particularly as all appropriate protocols have been met. However, she has suspicion (albeit based on little more than intuition) that the individual in question (possibly Teresa's husband) is presenting himself or herself to be a client when in fact he or she is not.

2. **Explore core issues and potential barriers to providing appropriate standard of care.** The primary concern is how best for Shanta to respond in the moment. Obviously she should refrain from discussing session content via text; however, it is unclear if she should make any additional efforts to contact Teresa using other means (e.g., request that she call her via videoconferencing to confirm her identity) or if she should just cease contact and wait until their next scheduled session to discuss the exchange in greater detail.

3. **Seek assistance/remediation for providing appropriate standard of care.** While Shanta should reach out for consultation from a supervisor or colleague with experience in distance counseling, this might not be immediately possible.

4. **Determine and evaluate possible courses of action.** Shanta has two options: Either she can try to contact Teresa using another means such as videoconferencing to determine her identity, or she can end contact at present and wait for their next session to discuss this matter in greater detail. If she declines to respond and waits until the next session to discuss further, she may be missing an opportunity to confirm not just Teresa's identity but also her well-being. While there is no substantive evidence that Teresa is in any immediate danger, the fact that her identity may have been compromised is concerning, and Shanta should do her best to confirm her client is in no immediate danger.

5. **Ensure that proposed actions promote client welfare.** Making efforts to verify Teresa's identity via voice or videoconferencing in the moment seems the most appropriate response. Shanta might also consider including in her informed consent a more detailed overview of the use of pass codes as an identity marker and what protocol will be followed if a data breach of some kind has occurred.

The Likely Answer

Shanta should discontinue the text messaging and make a telephone call to Teresa. If Teresa is unable to answer for any reason, Shanta should end ongoing contact until their next scheduled video session.

DISCLOSURE OF CONFIDENTIAL INFORMATION (*YOU GOT LISTSERVED*)

James is a second-year student in a professional counseling program who is currently completing his internship at a local college counseling center. One particular student, a senior nearing graduation, has been coming to see him weekly to discuss career plans following graduation. James offers a number of different recommendations to the student regarding plans after graduation, and he believes they have a strong rapport.

During this week's session, James is disheartened to note that the tone of their conversation is a bit awkward. The student, in a response that is surprising and frustrating to James, has disregarded his recommendations and tells James that they are irrelevant and unnecessary. James is unable to mask his annoyance at this response, and it becomes evident in session that he is disappointed with the student's reaction. After the session, the friction persists as James and the student engage in a flurry of email exchanges that are tense and leave James feeling disrespected. James seeks out time with his supervisor to discuss this interaction and his feelings of frustration. He spends the better part of an hour processing this with his direct supervisor, and he also has the opportunity to discuss this with other members of the counseling center staff.

After leaving for the day, however, James continues to feel agitated by this. He is part of a listserv community of counselors and opts to vent his frustrations further by posting a scathing commentary about his interactions with his client. The tone of this group is relaxed and casual, so James uses foul language and pejorative terms to write a stream-of-consciousness rant. He even posts a screenshot of one of the emails.

The next morning, James's supervisor contacts him via telephone. Several counseling students had approached faculty and reported being extremely uncomfortable with the nature and tone of James's statements about his client, but the main problem is that James accidentally posted his client's name and email address in the aforementioned screenshot.

Questions for Discussion

1. *How should James have dealt with his feelings about the client?*
2. *Is it ever acceptable for a counselor to process his or her feelings about a client on social media?*
3. *How should James's supervisor handle this situation?*

Straight From the Code

1. **H.6.d. Use of Public Social Media.** Counselors take precautions to avoid disclosing confidential information through public social media.

2. **B.7.b.** When consulting with colleagues, counselors do not disclose confidential information that reasonably could lead to the identification of a client or other person or organization with whom they have a confidential relationship, unless they have obtained prior consent of the person or organization or the disclosure cannot be avoided. They disclose information only to the extent necessary to achieve the purposes of the consultation.

Applying a Decision-Making Model: Kocet and Herlihy's CVCM (2014)

1. **Determine the nature of the value-based conflict.** James needed to remain calm in the face of clinical resistance and work through it with the client, asking questions and gathering information. This was a perfect opportunity to begin the decision-making process by James being candid about his surprise and conflicted feelings about the response that he was receiving from his client. Counselors should engage clients in discussions of challenges so that decisions regarding dilemmas can be made openly within the particular context of the relationship between the two parties. This level of candor may have also helped to give James a proper outlet for discussion and negotiation so that he did not feel the need to inappropriately express himself later.

   Counselors are expected to have negative reactions to clients at times, especially in the face of resistance; however, they need to maintain a basic level of professionalism, empathy, and respect for the client. Furthermore, confidentiality is a cornerstone of the counseling relationship, and each client should be able to rely on a counselor's commitment to it.

2. **Explore core issues and potential barriers to providing appropriate standard.** If James had been more mindful about the nature of this relationship, he would have remembered that he is the paraprofessional in this situation and needed to function in this manner. He needed to think about his responsibilities to the client, even at a time when being empathic was difficult. The client, while aware that James was being supervised, had every right to depend on James's professionalism and discretion. The client attended enough sessions to have an established relationship with James, and within that relationship, the client should have been able to expect confidentiality.

3. **Seek assistance/remediation for providing appropriate standard of care.** James did consult with colleagues regarding how to manage his frustration over the resistance he was receiving from the client. In fact, James consulted rather extensively. Not only did he have time to process with his direct supervisor, but he also had the opportunity to discuss with other colleagues how they handle this type of resistance. This support and advice was made readily available to James, and he appropriately took advantage of it.

   The ethics code is clear about maintaining client confidentiality. Section B.7.b. states, "When consulting with colleagues, counselors do not disclose confidential information that reasonably could lead to the identification of a client or other person or organization with whom they have a confidential relationship." James was entitled to consult with, and even vent wildly to, his colleagues regarding his experience of frustration with this client, and he could have done so without disclosing any identifying information about them.

4. **Determine and evaluate possible courses of action.** Clearly, the consultation and supervision he received failed to mitigate the level of agitation he experienced with his client. As previously mentioned, there was a fundamental disagreement with the client regarding James's recommendations. Had he given it some time and reflection, James could have processed this with his client in subsequent sessions and revisited it in supervision. Clients are entitled to disagree with their counselors, and counselors need to not feel threatened by this. Through the work, clients are given the opportunity to voice their opinions, and this would have been the perfect opportunity for James and his client to negotiate not only how recommendations are handled but also a mutually agreed-upon context of continued work. If consent could not be reached, arbitration remains an option. This could potentially be a role played by another member of the counseling center staff or James's direct supervisor.
5. **Ensure that proposed actions promote client welfare.** James's decision to disclose the client's identity, to reveal their email exchange, and to use such derogatory language when speaking about the client did not allow for reasonable consensus. Although the client never knew about the breach, eventually James's colleagues, supervisors, and peers from whom he sought consultation all knew. His choice put them in a position of having to report his unethical behavior to responsible parties and prohibited them from offering guidance, support, or alternative options to help him manage his emotions. If he had sought support in a different manner, he may have been able to get the type of consultation he needed to avoid the breach of confidentiality. His choice essentially required more direct action and consequences and eliminated the opportunity for further interactive reflection, negotiation, and consensualizing.

The Likely Answer

James's client should be made aware of the breach of confidentiality. James's supervisor should work with the colleague to determine a remediation procedure, and dismissal from the program should not be outside the realm of possibility.

IN-CLASS DISCUSSION AND EXERCISES

Group Discussion: Internet Presence

While it is inappropriate to look for information about clients using a web search engine, it is very likely that clients will look up their counselor. As such, being aware of your own Internet presence is important.

Take a moment and google your own name, making sure to use any iterations you may have used over the years. Is there anything in the search results that surprises you? Any images that are publicly available that you might not want clients to see?

Group Discussion: Confidentiality in the Social Media Age

Confidentiality is critical to the counseling profession, though technology adds another layer of complexity. While it is easier than ever to transmit information via technological advances, the risks to confidentiality are greater than ever.

In your current (or future) practice setting, what types of safety assurance measures are being utilized (or would make the most sense to utilize)? Is it objectively safe to use software programs for documentation and record keeping? How savvy are you (or the other clinicians in your practice) with regard to technology and the risks to client safety?

Role Play: Six Degrees of Separation

Using the scenario described in *Six Degrees of Separation*, role-play possible outcomes. Have one member play the role of Brendan and another play the role of Angela. If you were Brendan, how might you begin a dialogue? As Brendan, how might you actually feel or respond in the moment after one of your clients discusses your personal life without your consent? If Brendan were to express concern, how might Angela actually respond?

Documentation: Problem, Data, Assessment, and Plan

Using the Problem, Data, Assessment, and Plan (PDAP) format, pick one of the cases and write a progress note indicating the following:
Problem: What were the presenting concerns of this particular interaction?
Data: What, objectively, has happened? Remember to write this without subjective language or interpretation.
Assessment: As the counselor or supervisor in question, what *should* be done? Be sure to demonstrate comprehensive use of the decision-making model in this section.
Plan: What *will* be done? Be sure to outline a comprehensive plan that relates to the decision-making model.

References

American Psychological Association. (2019). *What you need to know before choosing online therapy*. Retrieved from https://www.apa.org/helpcenter/online-therapy

Education Amendments Act of 1972, 20 U.S.C. §§1681–1688 (2019).

Herlihy, B. J., Hermann, M. A., & Greden, L. R. (2014). Legal and ethical implications of using religious beliefs as the basis for refusing to counsel certain clients. *Journal of Counseling and Development*, *92*(2), 148–153. doi:10.1002/j.1556-6676.2014.00142.x

Kaplan, D., & Matz, E. (2014). Distance counseling, technology, and social media. *Counseling Today*. Retrieved from https://www.counseling.org/docs/default-source/ethics/ethics_sept_2014.pdf?sfvrsn=2

Kaplan, D. M. (2014). Ethical implications of a critical legal case for the counseling profession: *Ward v. Wilbanks*. *Journal of Counseling and Development, 92*(2), 142–146. doi:10.1002/j.1556-6676.2014.00140.x

Kocet, M. M., & Herlihy, B. J. (2014). Addressing value-based conflicts within the counseling relationship: A decision-making model. *Journal of Counseling and Development, 92*(2), 180–186.

Miller, W. R., & Rollnick, S. (2013). *Motivational interviewing: Helping people change* (3rd ed.). New York, NY: Guilford Press.

Nesmith, A. (2018). Reaching young people through texting-based crisis counseling. *Advances in Social Work, 18*(4), 1147–1164. doi:10.18060/21590

Remley, T. E., & Herlihy, B. (2019). *Ethical, legal, and professional issues in counseling* (6th ed.). Upper Saddle River, NJ: Pearson.

Shaw, H. E., & Shaw, S. F. (2006). Critical ethical issues in online counseling: Assessing current practices with an ethical intent checklist. *Journal of Counseling and Development, 84*(1), 41–53.

CHAPTER 9

RESOLVING ETHICAL ISSUES (SECTION I OF THE ACA CODE OF ETHICS)

INTRODUCTION

Though the American Counseling Association (ACA) Code of Ethics for professional counselors provides subsections for each area of practice related to clinical work and research, Section I engages in the more meta task of exploring how ethical dilemmas are actually resolved. In determining actions related to ethical dilemmas in their work with clients, the public, or other clinicians, counselors work to resolve these dilemmas with direct and open communication with all involved stakeholders. Counselors are required to know not just what the regulations of the profession are but also how best to uphold these regulations in their work.

All cases will be assessed using one of three separate decision-making models: Corey, Corey, Corey, and Callanan (2015), Cottone (2001), and Forester-Miller and Davis (2016).

PROTECTING CLIENTS FROM HARM: PART 1 (*NEWLY LICENSED COUNSELOR* REPORT-*ING FOR DUTY*)

Lucy is an in-home counselor working for a small facility in a rural area. She has been seeing a family for counseling over the past several weeks to address ongoing conflict following the son's recent involvement with probation. Due to a pending investigation (child welfare services had been notified of possible abuse by the mother), her services have been mandated by the state. The family is reluctant to participate, and the mother has stated on several occasions that she just wants to "get this over with and move on with our lives."

During today's session, the mother indicates that she had to break up a serious argument between her 13-year-old son, Jaron, and his 15-year-old sister, Liron. She states that she became upset during this altercation and slapped her daughter across the face. Liron and Jaron are both present during this discussion, and both laugh about it dismissively. However, scratches are visible on Liron's face from where her mother struck her.

Upon returning to the office, Lucy discusses the incident with her supervisor, Zoe. Zoe indicates it is "Lucy's call" as to whether she should report the incident, as it has been her experience that social services are less than helpful in this area.

If Lucy reports the incident, she risks losing rapport with the family. Additionally, services are already in place, which means that there is little the state would be able to do to provide help or support.

Questions for Discussion

1. *Does the act of slapping her child in the face out of anger and leaving marks constitute child abuse? Is Lucy obligated to file a report despite the fact that child welfare services are already involved?*
2. *Is there a way for Lucy to file this report that will* not *damage rapport with the family (and the mother in particular)?*
3. *Whether she decides to report the incident or not, how will Lucy work with the family moving forward?*

Straight From the Code

1. **I.2.c. Consultation.** When uncertain about whether a particular situation or course of action may be in violation of the ACA Code of Ethics, counselors consult with other counselors who are knowledgeable about ethics and the ACA Code of Ethics, with colleagues, or with appropriate authorities, such as the ACA Ethics and Professional Standards Department.

2. **A.4.a. Avoiding Harm.** Counselors act to avoid harming their clients, trainees, and research participants and to minimize or to remedy unavoidable or unanticipated harm.

3. **A.6.d. Role Changes in the Professional Relationship.** When counselors change a role from the original or most recent contracted relationship, they obtain informed consent from the client and explain the client's right to refuse services related to the change.

Applying a Decision-Making Model: Forester-Miller and Davis's Ethical Decision-Making Model

1. **Identify the problem.** In most states, corporal punishment of children is protected by law, and parents are free to use physical discipline (Knox, 2010). Many states are vague with regard to what constitutes corporal punishment versus abuse, typically differentiating by way of terms such as *unreasonable* or *excessive*. In Pennsylvania, for example, physical discipline is acceptable if it does not bring about "substantial risk of causing death, serious bodily injury, disfigurement, extreme pain, mental distress, or gross degradation" (Title 18, Section 509).

   Though it will be important for Lucy to determine the laws of her specific state, she must also recognize her responsibilities as a mandated reporter. A mandated reporter is any individual who may have frequent contact with children for whom it is required by law to report child maltreatment (National Clearinghouse on Child Abuse and Neglect Information, 2015), with *suspicion* of abuse alone meeting the criteria for a required report. Failure to report an incident of suspected abuse is a serious offense and can result in jail time in some states.

2. **Apply the ACA Code of Ethics.** The Code of Ethics has little to say about maltreatment of children and mandated reporting, presumably as this is specific to state law. A.4.a. makes clear that counselors avoid harming their clients but offers no specific guidelines related to mandated reporting. A.6.d. does indicate that Lucy needs to explain the change in her professional relationship (she is both evaluating for safety and providing counseling), though it is hoped that she made clear her responsibilities as a mandated reporter from the first meeting with the family.

3. **Determine the nature and dimensions of the dilemma.** There are three main concerns here. First, Lucy must determine if the mother's actions constitute abuse, and the laws in most states are vague in defining particulars. Second, whether the behaviors alone meet the criteria for abuse or not, Lucy must determine if this incident is enough to arouse suspicion as a mandated reporter that abuse of any kind is ongoing. Third, Lucy must determine what happens in her work with the family moving forward regardless of what choice she makes.

4. **Generate potential courses of action.** One possible option would be to immediately reach out to the family and be honest about her responsibilities as a mandated reporter. Lucy could highlight this as a matter of bureaucracy by saying that she has to do this to keep her job. This response would be honest in many ways but would ultimately undercut the severity of the incident. An anonymous report does not appear to be an option, as the family has only made Lucy aware of what has happened here.

   She could also simply choose not to file a report at this time and work with the family to develop anger management skills to be utilized during times of stress and interpersonal frustration. She could interpret the incident as an accident rather than an act of malice, in that the mother was acting in the interest of keeping her children from hurting one another. This, however, would also undercut the severity of the incident.

5. **Consider the potential consequences of all options and determine a course of action.** If Lucy does file a report, it seems very likely that this will damage her rapport with the family. It is hard to imagine that

the mother in particular would welcome another accusation that her parenting is abusive in some way. It also seems that her supervisor is probably right: Even if child welfare services in the area were *wonderful,* it is unlikely that anything other than mandatory in-home counseling would be assigned. Since this is what Lucy was doing with the family in the first place, it is doubtful that this would further the family's treatment in any significant way.

If, however, Lucy does *not* file a report, she puts her license (and in an extreme case, her freedom) in danger. For example, if the mother mentions the incident to child welfare services, resulting in an investigation where her behaviors in this case constituted abuse, Lucy could be in serious trouble. Worse yet, if this is actually part of a pattern of serious abuse that eventually results in more serious harm to these children, Lucy may have missed an opportunity to help.

6. **Evaluate the selected course of action.** Of the two options, reporting, and being honest with the family about doing so, seems the safest bet. In protecting the family, it ensures (as best she can) that a careful review of the events can take place and further support can be provided as needed. In protecting herself and her career, Lucy must remember that she will not be able to help any family or child if she loses her license (or is in jail).

7. **Implement the course of action.** Difficult conversations are never fun, but they are part and parcel to the counseling profession. Lucy will have to prepare herself to have a very honest talk with the entire family about why she has to make this choice.

The Likely Answer

Lucy should call the family back, ask to speak to the mom, and tell her she will be filing a report about what happened. After that, she has to do everything in her power to try and maintain rapport with the family and hope that they let her back in the house.

PROTECTING CLIENTS FROM HARM: PART 2 (*MENTAL HEALTH VS. PHYSICAL HEALTH VS. RELIGIOUS FREEDOM*)

Orcel is a school counselor working for a district in a rural area. Just after first period, Sonia, a 15-year-old sophomore, is brought to the school counselor's office by her teacher. Orcel is surprised to notice that Sonia's parents are accompanying her and that everyone looks visibly upset.

Sonia's teacher indicates that she had been acting "strange" for the past 4 days, as she had become unusually withdrawn and irritable in class. However, things escalated significantly today: At the start of class, Sonia appeared to have a petit mal seizure, during which she fell over at her desk and hit her head on the ground. She seemed to recover quickly but then locked herself in the faculty bathroom. She refused to come out until her parents showed up (whom she had apparently texted while in the bathroom), demanding to see their daughter.

Orcel meets with the parents privately while Sonia stays with the nurse. Her parents identify as Christian Scientists and state that they are averse to utilizing modern medicine based on religious principles. They explain that Sonia had never acted this way before but that she had recently suffered a "knock to the head" when she fell down the steps at home (which corresponds to 4 days ago, when her teacher noticed the behaviors began). They state that she reached out to them via text, as they instructed her to do if she needed someone to pray with.

The school nurse believes that these behaviors are consistent with a seizure disorder and notices that she has several contusions on her scalp. She recommends a follow-up with a physician and a psychiatrist, but her parents refuse. They are adamant that they will be heading home as a family, and the school cannot force them to seek medical treatment against their will. Sonia is present and cogent during this discussion and indicates that she agrees with her parents—she just wants to go home to pray.

Questions for Discussion

1. *Does the act of refusing medical care constitute child abuse? Is Orcel obligated to file a report?*
2. *Does the family's religious belief have any impact on the decision to file a report or not?*
3. *Does Sonia's age have any impact on the decision to file a report or not?*

Straight From the Code

1. **I.1.c. Conflicts Between Ethics and Laws.** If ethical responsibilities conflict with the law, regulations, and/or other governing legal authority, counselors make known their commitment to the ACA Code of Ethics and take steps to resolve the conflict. If the conflict cannot be resolved using this approach, counselors, acting in the best interest of the client, may adhere to the requirements of the law, regulations, and/or other governing legal authority.

2. **A.4.a. Avoiding Harm.** Counselors act to avoid harming their clients, trainees, and research participants and to minimize or to remedy unavoidable or unanticipated harm.

3. **A.6.d. Role Changes in the Professional Relationship.** When counselors change a role from the original or most recent contracted relationship, they obtain informed consent from the client and explain the client's right to refuse services related to the change.

Applying a Decision-Making Model: Forester-Miller and Davis's Ethical Decision-Making Model

1. **Identify the problem.** It seems highly likely that Sonia has a seizure disorder that requires further medical treatment, and a medical professional at the school has confirmed this. However, it is unclear if she or her parents are within their right to refuse medical care or if the school and its staff are obligated to intervene.

2. **Apply the ACA Code of Ethics.** As stated in the previous example, the Code of Ethics has little to say about maltreatment of children and mandated reporting, presumably as this is specific to state law. A.4.a. makes clear that counselors avoid harming their clients but offers no specific guidelines related to mandated reporting. A.6.d. does indicate that Orcel needs to explain the change in his professional relationship (he is both evaluating for safety and providing counseling), particularly as these concerns may not have been made clear if Sonia has never attended counseling before.

3. **Determine the nature and dimensions of the dilemma.** There are three main concerns here. First, Orcel must determine if Sonia meets the criteria as a child in the state in which this is occurring. For mental health treatment, the legal age of consent ranges from 12 to 16 years depending on the state (Kerwin et al., 2015). This means that Sonia would be considered an adult in the mental health system in Connecticut, but not in Kentucky. In Connecticut, she would be free to make her own choices, but in Kentucky, it would be her parents' decision (and their fault if she does not receive necessary care). Second, Orcel must determine if the referral is for a medical treatment or for mental health treatment, as state laws differ regarding age of consent. Most allow for consent to medical treatment at the age of 18 (McNary, 2014), which means that, if a seizure disorder is to be viewed as a medical treatment, it would again be her parents' decision and ultimate responsibility if she does not receive necessary care. Finally, Orcel must determine if an act of refusal to treat a medical or mental health condition that may result in serious injury constitutes abuse if the parents are adhering to a religious practice.

4. **Generate potential courses of action.** If the state where this occurs considers Sonia to be a child with regard to medical treatment but an adult with regard to mental health treatment, one possible option would be to inform the family of the need to file a report with child protective services and to do so immediately. In this case, it could be argued that the particulars are too convoluted and that allowing the state to decide is the safest alternative. If Sonia is considered to be an adult in the mental health system and Orcel believes that a

seizure disorder is more a mental health concern than a medical problem, another option might be to simply educate the family regarding treatment options and document the incident in its entirety. However, ignoring the organic components of a seizure disorder seems like a bit of a stretch in this case.

5. **Consider the potential consequences of all options and determine a course of action.** If Orcel does file a report, it is unclear if this will actually lead to better treatment for Sonia. If she is a child whose parents are refusing her medical care, it is unclear if a mandate of some kind will actually lead to Sonia receiving treatment or if the family will push back with litigation for infringement of religious freedom. However, there have been precedent-setting lawsuits that have addressed these matters. In *Commonwealth v. Twitchell*, it was established that parents do not have the right to deny their children access to medical care if it results in a possibility of serious harm or death (Margolick, 1990).

   If, however, Orcel does *not* file a report, he puts his license (and in an extreme case, his freedom) in danger. For example, if another educator present mentions the incident to child welfare services, resulting in an investigation where behaviors in this case constituted abuse, Orcel could be in serious trouble. Worse yet, if this is actually part of a pattern of serious abuse that eventually results in more serious harm to Sonia, Orcel may have missed an opportunity to help.

6. **Evaluate the selected course of action.** Of the two options, reporting, and being honest with the family about doing so, seems the safest bet. In protecting the family, it ensures (as best Orcel can) that a careful review of the events can take place and further support can be provided as needed. In protecting himself and his career, Orcel faces a similar concern mentioned in the previous case: He will not be able to help any child if he loses his license.

7. **Implement the course of action.** Time is of the essence here, as Sonia's health may be a serious problem that needs to be remedied quickly. Orcel must consult with the school and his direct supervisor before doing so if he is able, but he should likely be upfront with the family about his responsibilities as a mandated reporter while everyone is still in the same room.

The Likely Answer

Orcel should tell all family members about his duties as a mandated reporter, notify his supervisors at the school, make the report to child protective services, and hope everyone makes the right choice moving forward.

PREVIOUS RELATIONSHIPS AND COUNSELING (*HELLO FROM THE OTHER SIDE*)

Adele is a counselor in a drug and alcohol clinic. She sees approximately 25 clients each week for individual therapy and usually runs three group sessions in the early morning hours. For this particular program, clients are required to attend at least one group and one individual session weekly. The clinic (and its clients) are grateful that Adele is among the only clinicians willing to run these early hour meetings, as it allows working adults to get their required counseling hours without using sick time.

A new group of clients arrives for her 5 a.m. meeting: a psychoeducation group about mindfulness. Adele immediately recognizes one of the members in attendance is Alex, her high school boyfriend whom she has not seen or heard from since they broke up almost 10 years ago. Alex says hello and apologizes saying that he has been court ordered to attend these meetings and that Adele's is the only one he can attend without missing work. He asks if it would be okay to attend, promising that he will "not even acknowledge that we know each other."

Questions for Discussion

1. *Is it ever acceptable to treat a former partner or friend? Is 10 years long enough to justify that counseling Alex is acceptable?*
2. *If Adele does decide to treat Alex, how will she refrain from allowing their past relationship to interfere with counseling?*
3. *If Adele decides not to allow Alex to attend the group, what is she obligated to offer in its place?*

Straight From the Code

1. **I.2.d. Organizational Conflicts.** If the demands of an organization with which counselors are affiliated pose a conflict with the ACA Code of Ethics, counselors specify the nature of such conflicts and express to their supervisors or other responsible officials their commitment to the ACA Code of Ethics and, when possible, work through the appropriate channels to address the situation.

2. **A.6.a. Previous Relationships.** Counselors consider the risks and benefits of accepting as clients those with whom they have had a previous relationship. These potential clients may include individuals with whom the counselor has had a casual, distant, or past relationship. Examples include mutual or past membership in a professional association, organization, or community. When counselors accept these clients, they take appropriate professional precautions such as informed consent, consultation, supervision, and documentation to ensure that judgment is not impaired and no exploitation occurs.

Applying a Decision-Making Model: Forester-Miller and Davis's Ethical Decision-Making Model

1. **Identify the problem.** The primary problem is that Adele is in a position where she has either to deny a client a treatment that he or she needs or to treat a client with whom she has had a previous intimate relationship.

2. **Apply the ACA Code of Ethics.** The language in the code contains some ambiguity. Counseling clients from past relationships is discouraged, but not expressly forbidden; the language only states that counselors "consider the risks and benefits."

3. **Determine the nature and dimensions of the dilemma.** As with many ethical quagmires, a clear solution is not evident from the information presented or from the code. Adele will have to first consider the nature of her past relationship with Alex: Was the relationship brief or superficial such that a 10-year gap could suggest that counseling is plausible? Or was their relationship intimate in a way that would preclude objectivity? She would also have to consider the nature of the group: Is a psychoeducational group about mindfulness more education than counseling? Or is this a group that requires vulnerability and disclosure from its members?

4. **Generate potential courses of action.** The wording of the Code could allow Adele to take either path in this case. She could potentially justify that counseling is appropriate if the nature of the group is focused on education and her relationship with Alex was superficial in some way. She could also justify that having an ex-paramour as a client in any setting that constitutes counseling is wholly inappropriate.

5. **Consider the potential consequences of all options and determine a course of action.** If Adele decides to go ahead with treatment, she may be putting herself, Alex, and her clients in a difficult situation. Alex may know things about her that she would prefer not be shared with her clients, and she may know things about Alex that will mar her objectivity. If she decides not to treat him, she will have to be able to help Alex find reasonable accommodations such that he can be ensured of treatment elsewhere.

6. **Evaluate the selected course of action.** At present, it seems to make the most sense for Adele to not allow Alex to attend the group he has shown up for today. A decision such as this likely requires supervision, as she may run the risk of allowing her own biases to distort her perspective. Overconfidence in accuracy of decision-making among practicing clinicians can be a serious problem (Miller, Spengler, & Spengler, 2015), and clinicians should take care where personal biases might factor into the decision-making process.

7. **Implement the course of action.** If she meets with a supervisor and they collectively decide that Alex attending these groups is appropriate, she needs to be clear with herself, her supervisor, and Alex what constitutes acceptable boundaries given their unique circumstances. If not, they need to work together to find acceptable alternatives that meet Alex's needs.

The Likely Answer

Adele needs to tell Alex that it is wonderful to see him again (unless it is not) and that she needs to talk to her supervisor about next steps. It seems unlikely that she can justify having him in her group, though.

UNACCEPTABLE BUSINESS PRACTICES (*IS IT COOL IF WE KEEP SEEING EACH OTHER?*)

Marcy is a counselor at a private high school. As the school is small and values the reputation of its graduates, much of her time is spent working with graduating seniors to assist in the process of applying to colleges and universities. To say that these students are stressed is a bit of an understatement: Depression and anxiety are serious problems, as the pressure to succeed among the school's peer groups is *intense*.

Marcy has developed a strong rapport with Nick, a graduating senior who is planning on attending a very prestigious college an hour away from town. Nick has been struggling with tremendous anxiety related to his performance in college and is worried about starting over with a new counselor. On more than one occasion during their regular sessions over the past 2 years, he has said that Marcy is "the only counselor I've ever met who was able to offer any real help."

During their past meeting before the school year ends, Nick asks Marcy if it would be acceptable to continue meeting when he returns home for the weekends. He states that he already had a brief phone call with the counselor at his university but that he "just didn't like the sound of the guy." Though Marcy states that she does not do private practice work currently, he suggests that they could meet for individual sessions at the school on Fridays, as he knows her schedule and knows this is typically when she has an opening. He offers to pay her for her time.

Questions for Discussion

1. *Is it ever okay to accept a client for private pay work that was formerly a client at a salaried position?*
2. *Is it better to accept that Nick's concerns are valid or to encourage him to attempt establishing rapport with a new counselor at his university? In either case, what would need to be considered?*
3. *What would be the ethical concerns associated with seeing a former student during normal working hours?*

Straight From the Code

1. **I.1.b. Ethical Decision-Making.** When counselors are faced with an ethical dilemma, they use and document, as appropriate, an ethical decision-making model that may include, but is not limited to, consultation; consideration of relevant ethical standards, principles, and laws; generation of potential courses of action; deliberation of risks and benefits; and selection of an objective decision based on the circumstances and welfare of all involved.
2. **A.10.a. Self-Referral.** Counselors working in an organization (e.g., school, agency, institution) that provides counseling services do not refer clients to their private practice unless the policies of a particular organization make explicit provisions for self-referrals. In such instances, the clients must be informed of other options open to them should they seek private counseling services.
3. **A.10.b. Unacceptable Business Practices.** Counselors do not participate in fee splitting, nor do they give or receive commissions, rebates, or any other form of remuneration when referring clients for professional services.

Applying a Decision-Making Model: Forester-Miller and Davis's Ethical Decision-Making Model

1. **Identify the problem.** The main problem with Nick's suggestion is that Marcy does not have an established practice where she could see him. Seeing him for private pay might have been an option if this were the case, but using school property for independent business is likely a violation of her employment contract. Additionally, it is unclear based upon the information provided if this arrangement would be clinically sound, as it may be an indication of dependence as much as it is an indication of a good working alliance.
2. **Apply the ACA Code of Ethics.** The Code is thankfully clear on this matter, as referral to private practice is acceptable if it is in keeping with the standards of the organization (A.10.a). There is no indication of fee splitting, as the referral (if it were to happen) would ostensibly come from Marcy to herself.
3. **Determine the nature and dimensions of the dilemma.** It seems unlikely that the school would be willing to allow an employed counselor to meet with a former student for a private pay session on school grounds during working hours. It seems unlikely that Marcy would be able to find a way to continue seeing Nick unless she were to start her own private practice. Without this setup already in place, the dilemma becomes how best to ensure that Nick continues receiving help.

4. **Generate potential courses of action.** If Marcy felt strongly enough about her rapport with Nick, she could certainly reach out to administrators at school about her concerns (though again, this seems an unlikely resolution). Another option would be to work with Nick to address his anxieties about transitioning to a new therapist by asking him to sign a release to speak with his new clinician in the interest of facilitating a smoother transition. She could also offer phone support on a limited basis, as *booster sessions* such as these have been shown to have some benefit in other forms of counseling (Tolan, Gorman-Smith, Henry, & Schoeny, 2009).

5. **Consider the potential consequences of all options and determine a course of action.** Again, Marcy could certainly reach out to her superiors at the school if she felt strongly enough about Nick's concerns, but it seems highly unlikely that this would be determined to be a reasonable course of action. Periodic phone calls might be beneficial but could also easily facilitate dependence. Simply allowing for a *warm handoff* with his new counselor seems reasonable but could potentially make Nick feel a sense of abandonment per Marcy's refusal to continue treatment.

6. **Evaluate the selected course of action.** In this case, asking Nick to schedule an appointment with his new counselor and completing a release of information to discuss concerns regarding transition seems to be of lowest risk. If Nick begins this process and feels that the new counselor is not a fit for any reason, he can certainly work with Marcy to arrange a referral to another provider in the area that can accommodate him.

7. **Implement the course of action.** This will have to be managed carefully by Marcy, as her approach to ending treatment needs to be firm but compassionate in a way that honors Nick's perception of their time together. It seems very unlikely that there would be a way to continue seeing Nick that did not create either practical or ethical concerns, but Marcy still needs to be mindful of Nick's feelings and ongoing needs.

The Likely Answer

Marcy should be grateful that Nick valued their time together but will likely have to either offer a referral to an outpatient provider in the area or complete a release of information to speak with Nick's new counselor to aid in the process of transitioning.

DECEASED CLIENTS (*CONFIDENTIALITY SURVIVES DEATH*)

Kyra is a recent graduate of a professional counseling program who is currently working in a residential dual diagnosis treatment facility. She is being supervised by a licensed professional counselor and earning her hours for licensure. Kyra works independently with her full caseload of clients; however, she attends both individual supervision and group supervision with coworkers weekly, and she has wonderful rapport and trust with her supervisor.

When she arrived for work one day, Kyra was greeted with some tragic news: One of her clients passed away overnight. According to her supervisor who worked with the client extensively before Kyra, it was not an overdose but more likely the result of health issues neglected over the years. Kyra was very distraught at the news because her client was a wonderful man, with whom she had a delightful rapport. Kyra was quite optimistic about his recovery and felt they had made significant progress in their work together. While her coworkers handled her responsibilities for the day, Kyra spent extensive time in her supervisor's office receiving consultation and support. Kyra and her supervisor were also speaking to family members, who had, with the client's permission, been actively involved in his treatment. They were discussing details of the memorial service.

A few days later when Kyra was back to her regular responsibilities at work, she received a phone call from an upset woman claiming to be the estranged daughter of Kyra's client who had just died. The person on the phone was crying and screaming and angry that she had not been contacted and informed about her family member's death. Kyra became flustered and upset and wanted to help to calm the individual so, without much consideration, she began to discuss details of the situation with the caller. She told the caller of the circumstances as she knew them and also gave her information about the upcoming memorial services. After the phone call, Kyra was immediately unnerved, realizing that she had no way of knowing who was actually on the other end of the line. She remembered that her client had briefly mentioned a daughter, but she knew nothing more about her. The individual persisted in calling and attempting to gather more information over the next few days. Kyra was nervous and avoided her supervisor, the caller, and the client's family.

Questions for Discussion

1. *How should Kyra have handled the distraught individual that contacted her about her client?*
2. *What, if anything, should Kyra tell the caller?*
3. *What, if anything, should Kyra tell the client's family?*

Straight From the Code

1. **I.1.b. Ethical Decision-Making.** When counselors are faced with an ethical dilemma, they use and document, as appropriate, an ethical

decision-making model that may include, but is not limited to, consultation; consideration of relevant ethical standards, principles, and laws; generation of potential courses of action; deliberation of risks and benefits; and selection of an objective decision based on the circumstances and welfare of all involved.

2. **B.3.f. Deceased Clients.** Counselors protect the confidentiality of deceased clients, consistent with legal requirements and the documented preferences of the client.

Applying a Decision-Making Model: Cottone's Social Constructivism Model (2001)

1. **Obtain information from those involved.** Kyra reacted to this situation quickly and emotionally. If she had been in a different emotional state, and if she had thought about her basic duty of confidentiality to her clients, she would have responded to the caller by indicating that she could neither confirm nor deny that the individual about whom they were speaking was a client at the agency. Implementing the Cottone (2001) model, Kyra should have paused and taken the opportunity to begin gathering information that would help her to make an appropriate decision about how to handle this situation. The first step would have been to gather information about the individual on the phone. Even though she cannot rely on the caller to tell the truth, that would have been a start in the information-gathering process. Next, since the client had family that had been actively involved with his treatment for a long time, Kyra could have consulted with them, and with her supervisor, to gain a greater understanding of this person's relationship with the client. This would have helped to inform her decision-making process. Last, but perhaps most importantly, it would be essential to gain clarity about the client's desires with regard to this individual. A thorough review of the client's file would have been in order at this point.

2. **Assess the nature of the relationships operating at that moment in time.** Through the process of asking questions, Kyra would have spoken to her supervisor and discovered the contentious nature of the relationship between her client and the individual claiming to be his daughter. By reaching out to the family and determining the nature of their relationship with this person, she may have been better informed and prepared to make a decision. Through discussion with her supervisor, she would have learned that this individual was never previously involved with the client's treatment. The client's assertions to Kyra's supervisor that he did not want this person involved in his treatment would have been very useful information for Kyra to have.

3. **Consult with colleagues or the code of ethics.** The code of ethics is clear. Section B.3.f. states: "Counselors protect the confidentiality of deceased clients, consistent with legal requirements and the documented preferences of the client." Kyra needed to maintain the same level of confidentiality for her client in death that was maintained in life. The client's passing, while tragic and perhaps emotional for many people, does not change the parameters of confidentiality as he wanted them to be. Consulting with her supervisor or her colleagues, Kyra would have discovered the nature of the relationship between the client and this individual.

4. **Negotiate when there is a disagreement.** Typically, Cottone would call for negotiation and consensualization that involves the client at this point in an ethical dilemma; however, in this situation, while the client's interests are preeminent, unfortunately he is not available to advocate on his own behalf. In addition, the only area where there is disagreement is with the caller, and there is no room for negotiation here. Kyra erred in offering the caller any information at all because she was incapable of confirming the caller's identity and had no release permitting her to discuss the client's case with anyone other than the identified family members. Consensualization is Kyra's best choice at this point. Instead of avoiding the various people involved, Kyra needs to have open conversation with them to better understand their perspectives and opinions on the situation. Kyra is avoidant because of her mistake, but seeking guidance and insight and giving the family members the ability to express their informed and relevant opinions on the situation is crucial. Kyra should seek guidance from her supervisor on how to correct or minimize the impact of her misstep. She needs to inform the family of her mistake, so that they can be prepared for any potential consequences, and, she, along with her supervisor, need to develop a clear plan on how to deal with the persistent requests from the caller.

5. **Respond in a way that allows for reasonable consensus regarding next steps.** After talking to the involved family and reviewing the client's file, Kyra would have had a clear idea of where all parties stood in relation to the individual claiming to be the client's daughter. After consulting with her supervisor and reviewing the client's file, she would have been clear about the expectations placed on a professional in this situation. From there, Kyra could have made a decision reflective of a reasonable consensus among the stakeholders.

The Likely Answer

When Kyra received the initial phone call, despite the obvious emotional distress of the caller, she should have responded by neither confirming nor denying that the individual was a client at the agency. Now Kyra needs to be honest with the client's family about her initial misstep, as it may have a significant impact on them. In addition, she needs to be honest with her supervisor so that proper steps may be taken to handle accountability and any potential liability.

INTERDISCIPLINARY TEAMWORK (*WE'RE GETTING YOU OUT OF HERE!*)

Rose is a counselor who is working in a youth inpatient behavioral health hospital. Over the past few months, she has been working as the primary counselor for a 10-year-old client named Natalie, who was admitted earlier this year following serious behavioral disruption in the home.

During this week's treatment meeting, the team—the attending psychiatrist, Rose, and the other staff on the unit—collaboratively scheduled Natalie's discharge to a residential facility. This date was confirmed with Natalie's parents; however, Natalie herself has not yet been informed as she has a history of "self-sabotage" (i.e., increasing disruptive behaviors on the unit when she knows that a discharge is pending), and the team was trying to plan the best way of informing her.

A few hours after the meeting, Rose sees Natalie on the unit and asks her how she is doing. Natalie smiles and says, "Great! I'm going to a new facility next week." When Rose asks her how she knew about this, Natalie informs her that Daisy, another counselor on the unit who was also in the treatment meeting, told her all about it just a few minutes ago.

When Rose confronts Daisy about this, Daisy's response is simply to say, "Oh, that meeting was ridiculous. I've known this girl for months, and not telling her about something like this immediately is unconscionable!"

Questions for Discussion

1. *Did Daisy violate the code of ethics in any specific way?*
2. *How should Rose respond at this point? Should she tell the treatment team what happened or discuss this further with Daisy?*
3. *If Natalie was not a minor, would this situation be different?*

Straight From the Code

1. **I.1.b. Ethical Decision-Making.** When counselors are faced with an ethical dilemma, they use and document, as appropriate, an ethical decision-making model that may include, but is not limited to, consultation; consideration of relevant ethical standards, principles, and laws; generation of potential courses of action; deliberation of risks and benefits; and selection of an objective decision based on the circumstances and welfare of all involved.

2. **D.1.c. Interdisciplinary Teamwork.** Counselors who are members of interdisciplinary teams delivering multifaceted services to clients remain focused on how to best serve clients. They participate in and contribute to decisions that affect the well-being of clients by drawing on the perspectives, values, and experiences of the counseling profession and those of colleagues from other disciplines.

Applying a Decision-Making Model: Corey, Corey, Corey, and Callanan's Model

1. **Identify the problem or dilemma.** Despite having the best intentions, a counselor divulged information that was not hers to share. She did not technically violate the Code of Ethics related to confidentiality, but the hospital likely has very specific standards and a process in place for handling how patients are notified of changes in placement and/or progress.

2. **Identify the potential issues involved.** Regarding Natalie, there may be a direct impact on her well-being, as knowledge of her release has facilitated problems in the past. Regarding the inpatient unit in general, this might facilitate difficulties in reaffirming boundaries that are in place for patients and staff alike as well as create problems with consistency of care. Daisy's decision to discuss information with the patient that was previously only communicated by the primary counselor could result in poorly defined roles moving forward. Lastly, this could make the client lose faith in the staff, the primary counselor, and the facility due to their perceived communication struggles.

3. **Review the relevant code of ethics.** The concern in this case is teamwork within the healthcare setting. Daisy was clearly not behaving professionally as shown by disregard for her role on the team as well as her poor communication. She made a decision that was not agreed upon by the group, which only used her own perspective of the client.

4. **Know the applicable laws and regulations.** While Daisy's actions may not have violated any specific laws, it is highly likely that they went against organizational regulations. To best assist the patients by providing consistent structure, the hospital is likely to have set guidelines regarding how a discharge is supposed to be communicated.

5. **Obtain consultation.** At this point, Rose has to decide how to respond to this finding. It may be helpful for Rose to *table* her discussion with Daisy until she can speak with her direct supervisor. This meeting should likely take place very soon, as the impact on Natalie's treatment is imminent.

6. **Consider possible and probable courses of action.** Rose could first speak with Daisy about her actions and indicate her concerns, with

regard to both the ACA Code of Ethics and hospital policy. Another option would be to forego these discussions in favor of simply speaking with Daisy's and Rose's direct supervisor.

7. **Enumerate the consequences of various decisions.** If Rose only speaks with Daisy about her concerns, the problems regarding Natalie's treatment will not be resolved. If Rose goes over Daisy's head to her supervisor, the impact on workplace rapport may be substantial.
8. **Choose what appears to be the best course of action.** The best decision here would be a combination of the two of the choices. It would be helpful to clarify the situation with Daisy and also to reach out to Daisy's supervisor to explain the situation. An ideal outcome might be to treat the situation as a teachable moment and coachable opportunity. Ensuring that the entire staff, top to bottom, are on the same page with understanding their roles and boundaries will lead to more consistent care going forward.

The Likely Answer

Rose should express her concerns to Daisy, explain to her the need to discuss this with her direct supervisor, and then schedule a meeting with the treatment team to decide the next steps in Natalie's discharge plan.

POLICIES THAT ARE POTENTIALLY HARMFUL TO CLIENTS (*I OBJECT!*)

Francine is a school counselor in a large high school. At a weekly principal–counselors meeting with the high school administration, the building principal shares that the school counselors are now required to tell him when they suspect a student pregnancy, when a student reports a pregnancy, and/or when a student reports having or planning an abortion. This particular school has a history of having a high teenage pregnancy rate, one that is well above the national average.

Francine's supervisor, Debbie, is in attendance but does not say much, except that she would like to discuss the subject further with the principal privately at another time. Francine, however, is concerned about confidentiality and objects to the new policy that is being implemented. She is also angry this is being implemented without asking for the school counselors' perspectives. She worries that this policy will do more harm than good with how it is currently written and would like it to be reevaluated before implementation.

Despite how strongly she feels about this new policy, Francine is uncertain about vocalizing her concerns. She is aware that departmental politics can have a huge impact on contract renewals as well as salary increases.

Questions for Discussion

1. *Should Francine respond in the moment with her principal and other counselors present or should she first consult with the counseling department chairperson?*
2. *Is it appropriate for the principal to know about possible pregnancies and the outcomes as the administrator of the building?*
3. *Since this is now policy, what should the school counselors do now when they become aware of possible pregnancy?*

Straight From the Code

1. **D.1.h. Negative Conditions.** Counselors alert their employers of inappropriate policies and practices. They attempt to effect changes in such policies or procedures through constructive action within the organization. When such policies are potentially disruptive or damaging to clients or may limit the effectiveness of services provided and change cannot be affected, counselors take appropriate further action. Such action may include referral to appropriate certification, accreditation, or state licensure organizations, or voluntary termination of employment.

2. **D.1.i. Protection From Punitive Action.** Counselors do not harass a colleague or employee or dismiss an employee who has acted in a responsible and ethical manner to expose inappropriate employer policies or practices.

3. **I.2.b. Reporting Ethical Violations.** If an apparent violation has substantially harmed or is likely to substantially harm a person or organization and is not appropriate for informal resolution or is not resolved properly, counselors take further action depending on the situation. Such action may include referral to state or national committees on professional ethics, voluntary national certification bodies, state licensing boards, or appropriate institutional authorities. The confidentiality rights of clients should be considered in all actions. This standard does not apply when counselors have been retained to review the work of another counselor whose professional conduct is in question (e.g., consultation, expert testimony).

Applying a Decision-Making Model: Corey, Corey, Corey, and Callanan's Model

1. **Identify the problem or dilemma.** Francine would like to voice her concern about a new policy and the impact it will have on students, but she is also worried about the impact this will have on her employment. This policy was put in place without consulting the school

counselors or the department chair, and now the school counselors are responsible for implementing it.

2. **Identify the potential issues involved.** Francine may be correct in her assumption that she will face administrative backlash and a negative career impact for speaking up against a policy that is harmful and in direct opposition to her counselor training and understanding of confidentiality.

3. **Review the relevant code of ethics.** As a school counselor, Francine should refer to the American School Counselor Association (ASCA) Code of Ethics as well as the ACA Code of Ethics (refer to ASCA, 2018, position statement—*The School Counselor and Confidentiality*). Counselors should act in the best interest of their clients, and the implementation of a policy that purposely breaks confidentiality and could cause harm is likely unethical.

4. **Know the applicable laws and regulations**. It is important to know state laws regarding teen pregnancy as well as the school district's policy. The legality of confidentiality with regard to pregnant minors is complicated and can vary with regard to state and other factors (see Ott, 2014, for a detailed review).

5. **Obtain consultation**. In this case, it is evident that Francine's supervisor, Debbie, is already aware of the situation, since they were both in the same meeting together. As the department chair, Debbie has an obligation to discuss her concerns about this policy with the principal and share the outcome with the department. It would be beneficial for Francine to schedule a time to meet with her supervisor to express her concerns about both the policy and her fear of losing employment. It might be in the best interest of Francine or Debbie to survey the surrounding districts to see what their policies are.

6. **Consider possible and probable courses of action.** Scheduling a meeting with Debbie to process the meeting, the new policy, and how this impacts Francine as a school counselor is a possible solution. Another option would be for Francine to schedule a meeting with the principal directly. Francine could also do nothing at all and accept the policy for what it is.

7. **Enumerate the consequences of various decisions.** If Francine does nothing, this is likely to have a detrimental impact on her clients, and she has missed an opportunity to effect meaningful change in her district. If she meets with the principal, she is likely going over her supervisor's head, which may create conflict in the workplace.

8. **Choose what appears to be the best course of action.** Most likely the best course of action is where Francine meets separately with Debbie after reviewing the other school policies and referring to state law.

This is a proposal that will likely have a broad impact on the counseling services provided to students and is not a response that should be delivered independently by one counselor.

The Likely Answer

Francine should schedule a time to meet with Debbie privately to discuss her concerns about the new policy and her fears about the impact this will have on her clients. The two can work with the other counselors on staff to determine the best way to make their concerns known to the principal and related administration.

IN-CLASS DISCUSSION AND EXERCISES

Group Discussion: What Concerns You Most?

Practicing ethically is paramount to the success of the counseling profession. However, case examples such as those highlighted in this chapter demonstrate how complex the process of adhering to ethics can be, particularly when managing the needs of the client, the profession, the counselor, and any number of other potential stakeholders.

At this point in your training and/or practice, what are you most concerned about as potential *tripping points* in your work as a counselor? Difficulty maintaining confidence? Managing interpersonal conflicts? Navigating changes in technology?

Role Play: Newly Licensed Counselor...

Using the scenario described in *Newly Licensed Counselor...*, role-play possible outcomes. Have one member play the role of Lucy and another play the role of the mother. If you were Lucy, how might you begin a dialogue indicating that you may need to file a report of child abuse? As the mother, how might you actually feel or respond in the moment after your counselor indicated that they might have to file a report?

Documentation: Problem, Data, Assessment, and Plan

Using the Problem, Data, Assessment, and Plan (PDAP) format, pick one of the cases and write a progress note indicating the following:

Problem: What were the presenting concerns of this particular interaction?

Data: What, objectively, has happened? Remember to write this without subjective language or interpretation.

Assessment: As the counselor or supervisor in question, what *should* be done? Be sure to demonstrate comprehensive use of the decision-making model in this section.

Plan: What *will* be done? Be sure to outline a comprehensive plan that relates to the decision-making model.

References

American School Counselor Association. (2018). *The school counselor and confidentiality*. Retrieved from https://www.schoolcounselor.org/asca/media/asca/PositionStatements/PS_Confidentiality.pdf

Corey, G., Corey, M. S., Corey, C., & Callanan, P. (2015). *Issues and ethics in the helping professions* (9th ed.). Stamford, CT: Brooks/Cole.

Cottone, R. R. (2001). A social constructivism model of ethical decision-making in counseling. *Journal of Counseling and Development, 79*(1), 39–45. doi:10.1002/j.1556-6676.2001.tb01941.x

Forester-Miller, H., & Davis, T. E. (2016). *Practitioner's guide to ethical decision-making* (Rev. ed.). Retrieved from https://www.counseling.org/docs/default-source/ethics/practioner-39-s-guide-to-ethical-decision-making.pdf?sfvrsn=10

Kerwin, M. E., Kirby, K. C., Speziali, D., Duggan, M., Mellitz, C., Versek, B., & McNamara, A. (2015). What can parents do? A review of state laws regarding decision-making for adolescent drug abuse and mental health treatment. *Journal of Child and Adolescent Substance Abuse, 24*(3), 166–176. doi:10.1080/1067828X.2013.777380

Knox, M. (2010). On hitting children: A review of corporal punishment in the United States. *Journal of Pediatric Health Care, 24*(2), 103–107. doi:10.1016/j.pedhc.2009.03.001

Margolick, D. (1990). In child deaths, a test for Christian Science. *The New York Times*. Retrieved from https://www.nytimes.com/1990/08/06/us/in-child-deaths-a-test-for-christian-science.html

McNary, A. (2014). Consent to treatment of minors. *Innovations in Clinical Neuroscience, 11*(3–4), 43–45.

Miller, D. J., Spengler, E. S., & Spengler, P. M. (2015). A meta-analysis of confidence and judgment accuracy in clinical decision-making. *Journal of Counseling Psychology, 62*(4), 553–567. doi:10.1037/cou0000105

National Clearinghouse on Child Abuse and Neglect Information. (2015). *Mandatory reporters of child abuse and neglect*. Retrieved from https://www.childwelfare.gov/pubPDFs/manda.pdf

Ott, M. A. (2014). Teen pregnancy and confidentiality. *American Medical Association Journal of Ethics, 16*(11), 884–890. doi:10.1001/virtualmentor.2014.16.11.ecas3-1411

Tolan, P. H., Gorman-Smith, D., Henry, D., & Schoeny, M. (2009). The benefits of booster interventions: Evidence from a family-focused prevention program. *Prevention Science, 10*(4), 287–297. doi:10.1007/s11121-009-0139-8

INDEX